W9-DBE-686

# Tobacco Control

*Guest Editor*

NANCY L. YORK, PhD, RN, CNE

# NURSING CLINICS
# OF NORTH AMERICA

www.nursing.theclinics.com

*Consulting Editor*
SUZANNE S. PREVOST, PhD, RN, COI

March 2012 • Volume 47 • Number 1

SAUNDERS an imprint of ELSEVIER, Inc.

## W.B. SAUNDERS COMPANY

*A Division of Elsevier Inc.*

1600 John F. Kennedy Blvd., Suite 1800 • Philadelphia, PA 19103-2899

http://www.theclinics.com

**NURSING CLINICS OF NORTH AMERICA Volume 47, Number 1**
**March 2012 ISSN 0029-6465, ISBN-13: 978-1-4557-3898-4**

Editor: Katie Hartner
Developmental Editor: Donald Mumford

*Nursing Clinics of North America* (ISSN 0029-6465) is published quarterly by Elsevier Inc., 360 Park Avenue South, New York, NY 10010-1710. Months of issue are March, June, September, and December. Periodicals postage paid at New York, NY and additional mailing offices. Subscription price per year is, $144.00 (US individuals), $360.00 (US institutions), $260.00 (international individuals), $440.00 (international institutions), $210.00 (Canadian individuals), $440.00 (Canadian institutions), $79.00 (US students), and $129.00 (international students). To receive student/resident rate, orders must be accompanied by name of affiliated institution, date of term, and the signature of program/residency coordinator on institution letterhead. Orders will be billed at individual rate until proof of status is received. Foreign air speed delivery is included in all *Clinics* subscription prices. All prices are subject to change without notice. **POSTMASTER:** Send address changes to *Nursing Clinics*, Elsevier Health Sciences Division, Subscription Customer Service, 3251 Riverport Lane, Maryland Heights, MO 63043. **Customer Service: Telephone: 1-800-654-2452** (U.S. and Canada); **1-314-447-8871 (outside U.S. and Canada). Fax: 1-314-447-8029. E-mail: journalscustomerservice-usa@elsevier.com** (for print support) and **journalsonlinesupport-usa@elsevier.com** (for online support).

*Nursing Clinics of North America* is covered in *EMBASE/Excerpta Medica, MEDLINE/PubMed (Index Medicus), Social Sciences Citation Index, Current Contents, ASCA, Cumulative Index to Nursing, RNdex Top 100,* and Allied Health Literature and International Nursing Index (INI).

Printed in the United States of America.

# Contributors

## CONSULTING EDITOR

**SUZANNE S. PREVOST, PhD, RN, COI**
Associate Dean, Practice and Community Engagement, University of Kentucky, Lexington, Kentucky

## GUEST EDITOR

**NANCY L. YORK, PhD, RN, CNE**
Assistant Professor of Nursing, Bellarmine University, Lansing School of Nursing and Health Sciences, Louisville, Kentucky

## AUTHORS

**JACQUES (JACK) AMOLE, DNP, RN, PMHCNS-BC**
Assistant Professor, Department of Biobehavioral Nursing, Georgia Health Sciences University, College of Nursing, Athens, Georgia

**JEANNETTE O. ANDREWS, PhD, RN, FAAN**
Associate Dean and Professor, College of Nursing; Director, SCTR Center for Community Health Partnerships, Medical University of South Carolina, Charleston, South Carolina

**KRISTIN ASHFORD, PhD, APRN, RN**
Assistant Professor, University of Kentucky, College of Nursing, Lexington, Kentucky

**JOAN L. BOTTORFF, PhD, RN, FCAHS**
Professor and Director, Institute for Healthy Living and Chronic Disease Prevention, University of British Columbia, Kelowna, British Columbia, Canada

**KAREN M. BUTLER, DNP, RN**
Assistant Professor, College of Nursing; Faculty Associate, Tobacco Policy Research Program, University of Kentucky, Lexington, Kentucky

**BETTY JO CRAWFORD, RN, BSN**
Health Educator, Nevada Tobacco Users' Helpline, University of Nevada School of Medicine, Las Vegas, Nevada

**AUDREY DARVILLE, APRN, CTTS**
PhD Candidate, Certified Tobacco Treatment Specialist, Tobacco Policy Research Program, University of Kentucky College of Nursing; UKHealthCare, Lexington, Kentucky

**STEPHANIE DERIFIELD, MS**
Lawrence County Extension Agent, University of Kentucky, Louisa, Kentucky

**AMANDA FALLIN, PhD, RN**
Postdoctoral Fellow, Center for Tobacco Control Research and Education, University of California, San Francisco, San Francisco, California

**ELIZABETH E. FILDES, EdD, RN, CNE, CARN-AP**
Associate Professor, School of Nursing, Touro University Nevada, Henderson; Assistant Professor, Department of Psychiatry, University of Nevada School of Medicine, Las Vegas, Nevada

**ELIZABETH MORAN FITZGERALD, EdD, APRN, PMHCNS-BC**
Assistant Professor, Lansing School of Nursing & Health Sciences, Bellarmine University, Louisville, Kentucky

**DIANA P. HACKBARTH, RN, PhD, FAAN**
Professor and Program Director, Infection Prevention MSN & DNP, Niehoff School of Nursing, Loyola University Chicago; Project Director, School-based Health Center at Proviso East High School, Maywood; Co-Chair, Illinois Coalition Against Tobacco, Chicago, Illinois

**ELLEN J. HAHN, PhD, RN, FAAN**
Professor and Director, Tobacco Policy Research Program, Kentucky Center for Smoke-free Policy, University of Kentucky College of Nursing, Lexington, Kentucky

**REBECCA HAINES-SAAH, PhD**
Research Associate, School of Nursing, University of British Columbia, Okanagan Campus, British Columbia, Canada

**JAMES HAWKINS, MBA**
NFPG Practice and Compliance Manager, Department of Physiological and Technological Nursing, College of Nursing, Georgia Health Sciences University, Augusta, Georgia

**JANIE HEATH, PhD, APRN-BC, FAAN**
Associate Dean for Academic Programs and Professor of Nursing, University of Virginia School of Nursing, Charlottesville, Virginia

**SUSAN HEDGECOCK, MSN, RN**
Research Assistant, College of Nursing, University of Kentucky, Lexington, Kentucky

**WALLACE HENKELMAN, EdD, RN**
Assistant Professor, School of Nursing, Touro University Nevada, Henderson, Nevada

**SANDRA INGLETT, PhD, BSN**
Research Assistant, Department of Physiological and Technological Nursing, College of Nursing, Georgia Health Sciences University, Augusta, Georgia

**THOMAS V. JOSHUA, MS**
Instructor and Data Manager, Department of Physiological and Technological Nursing, College of Nursing, Georgia Health Sciences University, Augusta, Georgia

**SALOME KAPELLA-MSHIGENI, MPA, MPH**
Project Manager, Nevada Tobacco Users' Helpline, University of Nevada School of Medicine, Las Vegas, Nevada

**SARAH E. KERCSMAR, PhD**
Faculty Lecturer and Co-Director, Kentucky Center for Smoke-free Policy, University of Kentucky College of Nursing, Tobacco Policy Research Program; University of Kentucky College of Communications and Information Studies, Lexington, Kentucky

**KIYOUNG LEE, ScD, MPH**
Associate Professor, Tobacco Policy Research Program, Kentucky Center for Smoke-free Policy, University of Kentucky College of Nursing, Lexington, Kentucky; Graduate School of Public Health, Seoul National University, Gwanak-gu, Seoul, Korea

**MELISSA MCCANN**
Undergraduate Research Intern, Tobacco Policy Research Program, University of Kentucky College of Nursing, Lexington, Kentucky

**CAROLYN MCGINN, MS, RD**
Nutritionist and Health Educator, Lawrence County Health Department, Louisa, Kentucky

**BETH MCLEAR, MS, FNP-C**
Clinical Instructor, Department of Physiological & Technological Nursing, Georgia Health Sciences University, College of Nursing, Athens, Georgia

**DEBORAH MURRAY, EdD**
Associate Director, Health Education Through Extension Leadership, School of Human Environmental Sciences/FCS, University of Kentucky, Lexington, Kentucky

**SUSAN D. NEWMAN, PhD, RN**
Assistant Professor, College of Nursing, Co-Director, SCTR Center for Community Health Partnerships, Medical University of South Carolina, Charleston, South Carolina

**JOHN L. OLIFFE, PhD, RN**
Associate Professor, School of Nursing, University of British Columbia, Vancouver Campus, Vancouver, British Columbia, Canada

**RACHAEL A. RECORD, MA**
PhD Student, Tobacco Policy Research Program, Graduate Research Assistant, College of Nursing, University of Kentucky College of Nursing; University of Kentucky College of Communications and Information Studies, Lexington, Kentucky

**VIRGINIA HILL RICE, PhD, RN, CNS, FAAN**
Professor, Adult Health, Wayne State University College of Nursing and Karmanos Cancer Institute, Detroit, Michigan

**S. LEE RIDNER, PhD, APRN**
Associate Professor, School of Nursing, University of Louisville, Louisville, Kentucky

**CAROL A. RIKER, MSN, RN**
Associate Professor, Tobacco Policy Research Program, Kentucky Center for Smoke-free Policy, University of Kentucky College of Nursing, Lexington, Kentucky

**NITA SAKIEVICH, BA**
Clinic Coordinator, NFPG Tobacco Cessation Program, Augusta, Georgia

**GAYL SARBIT, PhD**
Knowledge Broker, Institute for Healthy Living and Chronic Disease Prevention, University of British Columbia, Okanagan Campus, Kelowna, British Columbia, Canada

**MARTHA S. TINGEN, PhD, APRN-BC**
Professor and Charles W. Linder Endowed Chair in Pediatrics, Department of Pediatrics, Medical College of Georgia, Georgia Health Sciences University, Augusta, Georgia

**SUSAN WESTNEAT, MA**
Epidemiologist, University of Kentucky, College of Nursing, Lexington, Kentucky

**CAMERON WHITE, PhD**
School of Nursing, University of British Columbia, Vancouver, British Columbia, Canada

**LOVORIA B. WILLIAMS, PhD, APRN-BC**
Assistant Professor, College of Nursing, Georgia Health Sciences University, Augusta, Georgia

**LISA A. WILSON, BS, MEd, CRCP**
Manager, UNR Office of Sponsored Projects, Las Vegas, Nevada

**MARTA A.T. WILSON, MS, MFT, CPC, LCADC, NCC, DCC**
Clinical Director, Division of Counseling and Prevention, Department of Psychiatry, University of Nevada School of Medicine, Las Vegas, Nevada

**SARA YOUNG, MD, MS**
Assistant Professor, Department of Family Medicine, Medical College of Georgia, Georgia Health Sciences University, Augusta, Georgia

# Contents

Nursing faculty practice groups can play a vital role in tobacco cessation in academic medical centers. Outcomes from the Georgia Health Sciences University Nursing Faculty Practice Group Tobacco Cessation Program revealed 64% abstinence outcomes at the end of treatment (N = 160) over a 2-year period from the campus-wide tobacco-free policy initiation. A nurse-led, evidence-based, interdisciplinary approach can be an effective strategy to make a difference in the lives of tobacco-dependent individuals, while at the same time integrating practice with education and research.

Prenatal exposure to secondhand smoke (SHS) is responsible for adverse perinatal outcomes, including preterm birth. Smoking at home is the primary source of exposure to women during pregnancy. Hair nicotine analysis of mothers and infants was used to describe the relationship between prenatal SHS exposure and number of household smokers. Maternal hair nicotine was strongly correlated with the number of household smokers and was a more sensitive measure of household smoking than infant hair. Home smoking bans and focused public media campaigns on the harmful effects of SHS exposure are necessary prevention strategies to avoid adverse perinatal outcomes.

Despite a strong stance by the American College Health Association and years of prevention and control efforts on US college campuses, smoking and exposure to secondhand smoke remain a problem among college students. This article provides an overview of what is known about cigarette smoking in this population as well as existing interventions for smoking prevention, cessation, and exposure to secondhand smoke on college campuses. Strategies to reduce tobacco use are presented, many of which have been demonstrated to be effective in the short-term.

Little is known about the most effective strategies to motivate rural smokers to quit. This article describes the personal narratives of current and former smokers living in an economically distressed, rural area of Appalachian Kentucky. Three categories emerged: personal motivators to quit smoking, external influences, pride of place. Capturing personal narratives represents an evidence-based, data-rich strategy for development of culturally sensitive, population-based interventions for rural smokers. Such strategies may be effective in reaching rural smokers and motivating them to quit, thereby reducing tobacco-related disease and premature death in rural, economically distressed communities.

Elizabeth Moran Fitzgerald

Pregnant Latina women living in the United States are a heterogeneous group represented by various countries, cultures, immigration status, and other socioeconomic factors. Although some of the literature refers to a Latina health paradox that may serve as a protective factor against smoking for recent immigrants, acculturation may increase the vulnerability of pregnant Latina women to begin smoking. Social-support treatments should be individualized based on what types of emotional, informational, or instrumental resources the woman desires. Evidence-based strategies delivered in English or Spanish by bilingual lay health educators and tailored to embrace Latina values are cost-effective and successful.

Joan L. Bottorff, Rebecca Haines-Saah, John L. Oliffe, and Gayl Sarbit

Smoking rates among and between men and women are in large part a reflection of the influence of gender and its intersections with other social factors including ethnicity, age, and social class that influence tobacco use and, ultimately, tobacco reduction and cessation. In this article, opportunities for developing and delivering gender-sensitive (programs addressing gender) and gender-specific (programs designed for men or women) interventions in the context of tobacco dependence treatment are discussed.

Jacques (Jack) Amole, Janie Heath, Thomas V. Joshua, and Beth McLear

This article presents an overview of an online education offering to improve standards of practice for nurses intervening with tobacco-dependent mentally ill populations. Designed as a pilot study and guided by the theory of reasoned action framework, the pretest-posttest educational program was conducted to examine attitudes and beliefs, knowledge, and intentions to integrate tobacco cessation interventions into practice. Although positive attitudes and beliefs were demonstrated, knowledge gaps continued to exist after the online program. Strengths and challenges of the online education offering are presented with recommendations for future research.

Jeannette O. Andrews, Susan D. Newman, Janie Heath, Lovoria B. Williams, and Martha S. Tingen

This article reviews the evidence of the use of community-based participatory research (CBPR) and smoking cessation interventions. An overview of

CBPR is provided, along with a description of the search methods and quality scoring. Research questions are explored to determine if CBPR improves the quality of research methods and community involvement in cessation intervention studies and cessation outcomes when using CBPR approaches. Results of the review are provided along with a comprehensive table summarizing all the included studies. Strengths and challenges of the CBPR approach are presented with recommendations for future research.

Tobacco use is the number one preventable cause of death and disability in the United States today. In 2003, the Interagency Committee on Smoking and Health recommended to establish a federally funded national tobacco quitline network by 2005. Quitlines are telephone-based programs that assist tobacco users to quit. The combination of health professionals referring patients to an accessible, evidence-based, cost-effective cessation resource can produce a substantial reduction in the number of tobacco users in the United States. Initiatives to increase knowledge and working relationships between nurses and quitlines need to be created, implemented, and evaluated.

**Section II: Policy Advances for Tobacco Control**

This article describes a 3-pronged compliance strategy to implement a tobacco-free campus policy at 1 large, land grant public university in the South, and evaluates its impact on outcomes and costs. Although there has been a recent wave of tobacco-free colleges, policy restrictiveness and implementation vary, and compliance remains a challenge. The 3 Ts strategy (Tell-Treat-Train) involves regular, consistent communications, access to tobacco treatment medications and counseling, and ongoing training of supervisors and student leaders. Administrative support, access to tobacco treatment, campus buy-in, sustained communications, and careful implementation planning are critical to instituting a tobacco-free university policy.

Tobacco use among adolescents is declining in the United States but remains a major public health problem in the United States and globally. The Healthy People 2020 model of determinants of health is useful in understanding the complex interaction of factors that help explain adolescent smoking-related behaviors. Nurses are well positioned to take leadership roles in health care settings, schools, and their own communities as well as at the state, national, and global levels in advocating for

## FORTHCOMING ISSUES

*June 2012*
**Future of Advanced Nursing Practice**
Robin Dennison, DNP, MSN, CCNS, RN,
*Guest Editor*

*September 2012*
**Second Generation Work with QSEN**
Joanne Disch, PhD, RN, FAAN, and
Jane H. Barnsteiner, PhD, FAAN,
*Guest Editors*

*December 2012*
**New Developments in Nursing Education**
Mary Ellen Smith Glasgow, PhD, RN,
ACNS-BC, *Guest Editor*

## RECENT ISSUES

*December 2011*
**Victims of Abuse**
Sharon W. Stark, PhD, RN, APN-C, CFN,
*Guest Editor*

*September 2011*
**Patient Education**
Stephen D. Krau, PhD, RN, CNE,
*Guest Editor*

*June 2011*
**Culturally Competent Care**
Diane B. Monsivais, PhD, CRRN,
*Guest Editor*

## THE CLINICS ARE NOW AVAILABLE ONLINE!

Access your subscription at:
**www.theclinics.com**

# Preface

# Tobacco Use and Control in the United States

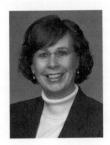

Nancy L. York, PhD, RN, CNE
*Guest Editor*

Tobacco use remains the leading cause of preventable death in the United States despite numerous advances in tobacco prevention and control within the past two decades. Although smoking prevalence rates are declining as a result of these efforts, the Centers for Disease Control and Prevention (CDC) estimates 46 million, or 20.6%, adults in the United States smoke cigarettes.[1] The CDC also estimates 1 in 5 deaths in the United States is attributable to cigarette smoking[2] and that, on average, adult cigarette smokers will die 14 years earlier than nonsmokers.[3]

Researchers have unequivocally linked smoking with multiple forms of cancer, cardiovascular diseases, pulmonary diseases, fertility issues, and damaging developmental effects.[4] Additionally, secondhand smoke (SHS), which includes smoke from the end of a burning cigarette, cigar, or pipe, combined with smoke exhaled by the smoker, is also indisputably related to increased risk of lung cancer and heart disease in adults, and ear infections, asthma attacks, respiratory infections, and sudden infant death syndrome in infants and children.[5]

The economic costs related to smoking are staggering as well. Smokers spend approximately $83.6 billion on cigarettes[6] and $2.6 billion on smokeless tobacco products[7] annually in the United States. Smoking-related diseases result in more than $96 billion in direct health care costs, while it is estimated that $97 billion is lost in productivity annually.[8]

As cigarette smoking has become less socially acceptable in the United States, the tobacco industry has changed their advertising focus to other markets, including developing countries, alternative tobacco products, and targeting younger smokers. Today tobacco can be consumed by methods other than cigarette smoking, including chewing tobacco, moist snuff, snus, pellets, electronic cigarette devices, cigar and pipe smoking, and hookah use. Many of these alternative products are being targeted at younger smokers who are the most susceptible to marketing and advertising strategies.[9,10]

Nurs Clin N Am 47 (2012) xiii–xiv
doi:10.1016/j.cnur.2011.10.012
0029-6465/12/$ – see front matter © 2012 Elsevier Inc. All rights reserved.

nursing.theclinics.com

This issue of *Nursing Clinics of North America* outlines the amazing work of nurses related to tobacco control. The issue begins with a detailed review of cessation efforts offered to various populations in the United States and Canada. Researchers have found that evidence-based targeted cessation programs are the most effective way to improve adherence to cessation therapies and decrease smoking prevalence rates. Second, given that tobacco use is now viewed as a population issue versus an individual behavior, this issue also discusses policy advances to protect communities from involuntary exposure to SHS. Studies have shown smoke-free policies lead to decrease smoking prevalence rates and improve smoker cessation efforts. Finally, the authors discuss popular tobacco products currently being targeted at younger smokers.

Nancy L. York, PhD, RN, CNE
Bellarmine University
Lansing School of Nursing & Health Sciences
2001 Newburg Road, Miles Hall 201
Louisville, KY 40299, USA

E-mail address:
nyork@bellarmine.edu

**REFERENCES**

1. Centers for Disease Control and Prevention. Vital signs: Current cigarette smoking among adults aged >18 years—United States, 2009. Morbid Mort Wkly Rep 2010;59(35):1135–40.
2. Centers for Disease Control and Prevention. Smoking-attributable mortality, years of potential life lost, and productivity losses—United States, 2000-2004. MMWR Morb Mortal Wkly Rep 2008;57(45):1226–8.
3. Centers for Disease Control and Prevention. Annual smoking-attributable mortality, years of potential life lost, and economic costs—United States, 1995-1999. MMWR Morb Mortal Wkly Rep 2002;51(14):300–3.
4. Centers for Disease Control and Prevention. Smoking and Tobacco Use. Health Effects. Available at: http://www.cdc.gov/tobacco/basic_information/health_effects/index.htm. Accessed October 13, 2011.
5. Centers for Disease Control and Prevention. Smoking and Tobacco Use. Secondhand Smoke (SHS) Facts. Available at: http://www.cdc.gov/tobacco/data_statistics/fact_sheets/secondhand_smoke/general_facts/index.htm. Accessed October 13, 2011.
6. U.S. Department of Agriculture. Expenditures for Tobacco Products and Disposable Personal Income, 1989-2006. Washington, DC: U.S. Department of Agriculture, Economic Research Service; 2007.
7. Federal Trade Commission Smokeless Tobacco Report for the Year 2009. Available at: http://www.ftc.gov/os/2009/08/090812smokelesstobaccoreport.pdf. Accessed October 13, 2011.
8. U.S. Department of Agriculture. Briefing Room: Tobacco—Background. Washington, DC: U.S. Department of Agriculture, Economic Research Service; 2005.
9. MacKintosh AM, Moodie C, Hastings G. The association between point-of-sale displays and youth smoking susceptibility. Nicotine Tobacco Res 2011. [Epub ahead of print].
10. DiFranza JR, Wellman RJ, Sargent JD, et al. Tobacco promotion and the initiation of tobacco use: assessing the evidence for causality. Pediatrics 2006;117(6):1237–48.

# The Impact of the Georgia Health Sciences University Nursing Faculty Practice on Tobacco Cessation Rates

Janie Heath, PhD, APRN-BC[a],*, Sandra Inglett, PhD, BSN[b],
Sara Young, MD, MS[c], Thomas V. Joshua, MS[b], Nita Sakievich, BA[d],
James Hawkins, MBA[b], Jeannette O. Andrews, PhD, RN[e],
Martha S. Tingen, PhD, APRN-BC[f]

**KEYWORDS**

- Tobacco cessation • Nursing faculty practice
- Evidence-based practice

Academic health centers expend considerable time and resources in preventing and treating illness and injury, as well as promoting healthy lifestyles. The trend toward tobacco-free environments is growing nationwide and positions academic centers to reinforce the health commitment to employees, students, and the community. Although the prevalence of smoking in Georgia has decreased from 32% to 20% of the state's population over the past 20 years, far too many Georgians, 1 out of 5, continue to smoke. In addition, more than a third of Georgia's children live with individuals who smoke, and each year 11,000 Georgians die prematurely from smoking

---

The authors have no financial disclosures and/or conflicts of interest to disclose.
[a] University of Virginia School of Nursing, Claude Moore Nursing Education Building, PO Box 800826, 225 Jeanette, Lancaster Way, Charlottesville, VA 22908-0826, USA
[b] Department of Physiological and Technological Nursing, College of Nursing, Georgia Health Sciences University, 987 Saint Sebastian Way, EC 5426, Augusta, GA 30912, USA
[c] Department of Family Medicine, Medical College of Georgia, Georgia Health Sciences University, 1120 15th Street, Augusta, GA 30912, USA
[d] NFPG Tobacco Cessation Program, 987 Saint Sebastian Way, EC 5396, Augusta, GA 30912, USA
[e] College of Nursing, Medical University of South Carolina, 99 Jonathan Lucas Street, MSC 160, Charleston, SC 29425, USA
[f] Department of Pediatrics, Medical College of Georgia, Georgia Health Sciences University, 1120 15th Street BT 1852, Augusta, GA 30912, USA
* Corresponding author.
*E-mail address:* Janie.heath@virginia.edu

or exposure to secondhand smoke.[1,2] Nationally, the annual death toll from tobacco use approaches 450,000, surpassing combined deaths due to alcohol, car accidents, suicides, homicides, human immunodeficiency virus disease, and illicit drug use.[3] For every death attributable to smoking or exposure to secondhand smoke, the Centers for Disease Control and Prevention estimates that 20 other people are living with a tobacco-related illness such as cancer, heart disease, or emphysema.[4]

Recognizing that the numbers are too staggering to be silent, the Georgia Health Sciences University (GHSU) enterprise (academic units, clinical services, and physician practice group) made an administrative decision to become tobacco free. As Georgia's only health sciences university and the Central Savannah River Area's only academic medical center, GHSU undertook the initiative to be a leader in protecting employees, students, patients, and visitors from the harmful effects of secondhand smoke. Driven by the GHSU mission, "to improve health and reduce the burden of illness in society," in August, 2006, a task force of more than 40 representatives from the university, hospital, and clinics worked for more than a year to implement a plan for a smooth transition to becoming a tobacco-free environment.[5]

## BACKGROUND

After 15 months of committee work, GHSU's goal to become a tobacco-free campus became a reality on November 17, 2007, the 31st anniversary of the American Cancer Society's Great American Smokeout. Another significant goal with the tobacco-free initiative was a partnership with the GHSU College of Nursing (CON). Under the auspices of the College of Nursing Faculty Practice Group (NFPG), the GHSU Tobacco Cessation Clinic was approved to be the exclusive provider of free tobacco cessation treatment services for patients, students, and employees. Although the authors of this article are not aware of a nursing faculty practice model for tobacco cessation in the workplace setting reported in the literature, a systematic review of 26 studies investigating the effects of smoking bans in the workplace found that smoking bans led to a 3.8% reduction in the prevalence of smokers among employees. Furthermore, those employees who continued to smoke averaged 3.1 fewer cigarettes per day.[6]

Established in 2006, the NFPG integrates clinical practice, education, and research through faculty practice activities that promote high-quality cost-effective health care and access to care with the following purposes:

1. To further the service, education, and research missions of the GHSU and the University System of Georgia Board of Regents
2. To enable faculty to maintain clinical competence, fulfill certification requirements, and share expertise with other health care providers
3. To provide additional revenue streams for the CON and salary supplementation for the faculty members.[7]

The Tobacco Cessation Clinic is a patient/family-centered clinic facilitated by certified advanced practice nurses with more than 50 years of combined clinical and tobacco cessation experience. Located in the 350 m$^2$ GHSU Interdisciplinary Practice and Research Center in the CON and College of Allied Health Sciences Building, the clinic provides cessation services to employees, students, and community residents.[8] Members of the NFPG Tobacco Cessation Clinic team (**Fig. 1**) include a practice manager, a clinic administrative assistant, clinical nurse specialists, nurse practitioners, biobehavioral and nurse researchers, respiratory therapists, a clinical pharmacist, and a primary care physician. Similar to other nursing faculty practice models, the mission of the NFPG Tobacco Cessation Clinic values integration of practice with

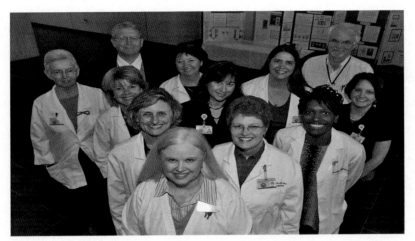

Fig. 1. Tobacco cessation team.

education and research.[9–12] Unique to the faculty practice model is the opportunity for interprofessional learning among students in allied health sciences, pharmacy, and nursing to make a difference in tobacco-dependent populations.

Recognized as an interdisciplinary centerpiece for providing clinical services and training site opportunities, advanced practice nurse members of the NFPG Tobacco Cessation Clinic apply evidence-based strategies of the United States Public Health Service (USPHS) Guideline for Treating Tobacco Dependence.[8,13] With year-round services, the NFPG Tobacco Cessation Clinic provides the following treatment options:

- Weekly group sessions for 6 weeks, weekly individual sessions for 4 weeks, or combination of group and individual sessions
- All treatment sessions include
  - Prescreening (medical evaluation by a nurse practitioner)
  - Weekly monitoring of carbon monoxide, blood pressure, heart rate, and weight
  - Weekly assessment of tobacco use, readiness to quit, and confidence to quit
  - Strategies to help smokers quit
  - Nicotine addiction and emotional dependence overview
  - Social support, coping strategies, and stress management
  - Nicotine replacement therapies and other pharmacotherapy agents
  - Triggers to smoke and problem-solving skills
  - Cognitive/behavioral strategies
  - Weight control
  - Relapse prevention
  - Telephone follow-up at 3 months, 6 months, and 12 months.

Budgetary requirements for the NFPG Tobacco Cessation Clinic business proposal were partially based on the enterprise-wide survey conducted with approximately 10,000 GHSU students, faculty, and classified employees. Thirty percent of the campus responded; 12.8% reported a positive current smoker status and more than 47% reported smoking 1 to 2 packs per day. In addition, approximately 1000 patients, families, and visitors were surveyed during that time, and 27% reported current tobacco use.[5] These data supported the campus decision to cover $655 costs per employee and/or student during a 2-year period for free tobacco cessation treatment, covering both behavioral counseling ($285) and pharmacotherapy costs ($370).

## PROGRAM PROCEDURES

Practice agreements for the NFPG Tobacco Cessation Clinic's advanced practice nurses (nurse practitioners and clinical nurse specialists) were first approved by the GHSU credentialing committee. Based on the USPHS guideline for treating tobacco dependence, which recommends a combination of tobacco cessation counseling and pharmacotherapy be provided to maximize effectiveness of cessation efforts,[13] a GHSU primary care physician (S.Y.) agreed to be the collaborating medical director for the clinic. All advanced practice nurses and allied health providers (respiratory therapists) who facilitated group or individual counseling sessions were certified and/or trained as tobacco cessation specialists or facilitators. The clinic materials for behavioral counseling were predominantly from the American Lung Association's Freedom from Smoking[14] and customized NFPG Tobacco Cessation Clinic materials from the Nurses for Tobacco Control Coalition (NTCC) Web site.[15]

As academic nurse leaders for the NTCC (J.H., S.I.), the NFPG Tobacco Cessation Clinic directors used the REAP (research, education, advocacy, and practice) framework to facilitate activities for student integration and infrastructure to support scholarly activities.[15] More than 30 undergraduate nursing students (bachelor of science in nursing) and graduate nursing students (master of science in nursing–certified nurse leader, nurse practitioner, doctorate in nursing practice, and doctor of philosophy) were integrally involved, as well as respiratory therapy and pharmacy students, with the NFPG Tobacco Cessation Clinic sessions. The GHSU Human Assurance Committee approved the program procedures, and participants signed informed consents during the baseline assessment session (medical evaluation/clearance). Business agreements were established with a local pharmacy to serve as a partner for providing tobacco cessation pharmacologic aids.

Multiple venues were used to promote the free services of the NFPG Tobacco Cessation Clinic as the Tobacco-Free Campus initiative unfolded. The predominant means of communication was through the *GHSU Beeper* (newsletter) and e-blasts. Participants were eligible for the clinic and follow-up survey if they were older than 18 years, smoked at least 1 cigarette daily, and were motivated to quit smoking within the first 30 days of the clinic. All participants received a tobacco history (including Fagerström Test for Nicotine Dependence), medical history, and brief physical assessment at baseline by NFPG nurse practitioners. Biological measures, such as carbon monoxide level, blood pressure, heart rate, and weight, were obtained at baseline and assessed weekly. Participants self-selected either group session counseling for 6 weeks or individual session counseling for 4 weeks. Each of the counseling sessions lasted approximately 2 hours. Most group sessions were conducted on either a Monday morning (10 AM–12 PM) or Thursday evening (5 PM–7 PM). Individual sessions were reserved for participants with employee schedule conflicts or mental health conditions. Most counseling sessions were provided by NFPG clinical nurse specialists with psych-mental health expertise.

Pharmacotherapy options were discussed with each participant individually during the baseline assessment by a nurse practitioner and reviewed again during the counseling session for the risks and benefits of nicotine replacement therapy, bupropion, and/or varenicline. Through mutual agreement about the medication of choice, prescriptions were either telephoned or faxed to the pharmacy partner before the second clinic session, and each participant received a 12-week supply. Doses for tobacco cessation pharmacotherapy aligned with each product's prescribing information, and if any concerns were identified, the pharmacotherapy options were discussed with the participant's primary care provider and/or NFPG Tobacco Cessation Clinic medical director.

All participants were required to complete the 20-item Center for Epidemiological Studies-Depression (CES-D) instrument as baseline to assess for mental health concerns. The NFPG practice agreement included a score of 20 or more on the CES-D scale to be of concern for varenicline use and designated other pharmacotherapy options to be explored and/or consultation sought with the primary care provider or the clinical medical director. In addition, all positive medical histories of potential renal impairment conditions, such as hypertension or diabetes, required serum creatinine evaluation before varenicline use.

## PROGRAM OUTCOMES

From November 2007 to November 2009, enrollment in the NFPG Tobacco Cessation Clinic included 160 participants, of whom 147 received free treatment as GHSU employees/students; 13 community members enrolled for a fee. Outcomes for analyses included end-of-treatment abstinence rates (4-week treatment for individual sessions or 6-week treatment for group sessions) at 3 months (telephone and/or e-mail), 6 months (telephone and/or e-mail), and 12 months (telephone and/or e-mail). All end point analyses were based on a 7-day point prevalence for self-reports on tobacco cessation. End-of-treatment self-report outcomes (group, 6 weeks; individual, 4 weeks) were validated with carbon monoxide readings. All participants lost to follow-up were coded as smokers.

Of the 160 participants enrolled for treatment, most were women (55%), and the average age was 42.3 years (standard deviation [SD] = 10.9), with a range of 21 to 71 years (**Table 1**). The participants included 92% GHSU employees and/or students and 8% community members. Sixty-five percent (N = 104) had college degrees or attended some college; the remainder had General Education Development, high school, or vocational training. Most participants reported smoking cigarettes (94.3%); the remaining participants either smoked cigars (3.7%) or used smokeless tobacco (6.8%). Five percent of the participants (N = 8) reported polytobacco use. Ninety-five percent of the participants had made at least 1 serious attempt to quit before enrollment in the NFPG tobacco cessation program, with 48% trying to quit cold turkey.

Eighty-six percent (N = 138) of the participants attended group sessions and the remaining participants (N = 22) attended individual sessions. At baseline, the participants had an average Fagerström nicotine dependence score of 4.4 (SD = 1.8) on a scale of 1 to 10, a daily cigarette use of 16.8 (SD = 9.0), a readiness-to-quit scale average of 7.4 on a scale of 0 to 10, and an average CES-D score of 12.6 on a scale of 0 to 60, with 16 to 26 indicating mild depression. Over the baseline and end-of-treatment period, carbon monoxide levels (**Table 2**) reduced by 37% and weight increased by 1.3% (average, 1.1 kg [2.5 lb]). Systolic, diastolic, and heart rate remained relatively stable.

Ninety-one percent (N = 145) of the participants received medication: 11% received nicotine replacement therapy (N = 6 patch, N = 3 gum, N = 5 lozenge, N = 2 inhaler) as monotherapy or combination therapy; 97.9% received non–nicotine replacement therapy, either sustained-released bupropion (N = 4) or varenicline (N = 138). 9.4% (N = 15) of participants did not use pharmacotherapy. Overall, 69% of participants on pharmacotherapy reported at least 1 side effect during treatment. Forty-nine

| Table 1 Baseline participant characteristics and smoking history (N = 160[a]) | | |
|---|---|---|
| **Characteristics** | **n** | **(%)** |
| Gender | | |
|   Women | 88 | (55.0) |
|   Men | 72 | (45.0) |
| Ethnicity | | |
|   African American | 29 | (18.2) |
|   Caucasian | 125 | (78.6) |
|   Asian | 4 | (2.5) |
|   Other | 1 | (0.6) |
| Age (y) | | |
|   Mean (SD) | 42.3 | (10.9) |
|   Range | 21–71 | — |
| Marital status | | |
|   Married | 84 | (52.5) |
|   Single | 44 | (27.5) |
|   Divorced | 24 | (15.0) |
|   Other | 8 | (5.4) |
| Education | | |
|   College degree/attended | 104 | (65.0) |
|   High school/General Education Development/technical training | 45 | (28.1) |
| Years of tobacco use | | |
|   Mean (SD) | 23.8 | (11.7) |
|   Range | 0.8–62 | — |
| Type of tobacco use | | |
|   Cigarettes | 151 | (94.4) |
|   Cigar | 6 | (3.8) |
|   Smokeless tobacco | 11 | (6.9) |
| Number of cigarettes smoked per day | | |
|   Mean (SD) | 16.8 | (9.0) |
|   Range | 1–80 | — |
| Type of quit attempts | | |
|   Cold turkey | 73 | (48.3) |
|   Counseling | 4 | (2.7) |
|   Alternative (hypnosis/acupuncture) | 7 | (4.7) |
|   NRT patch | 43 | (28.5) |
|   NRT gum | 20 | (13.3) |
|   NRT lozenge | 8 | (5.3) |
|   NRT inhaler | 4 | (2.6) |
|   Bupropion | 16 | (10.6) |
|   Varenicline | 17 | (11.3) |
| Fagerström nicotine dependence | | |
|   Mean (SD) | 4.4 | (1.8) |
|   Range | 1–10 | — |

*(continued on next page)*

| Table 1 (continued) | | |
|---|---|---|
| Characteristics | n | (%) |
| CES-D | | |
| Mean (SD) | 12.6 | (8.2) |
| Range | 1–42 | — |
| Readiness to quit | | |
| Mean (SD) | 7.4 | (1.0) |
| Range | 1–10 | — |

*Abbreviation:* NRT, nicotine replacement therapy.
[a] Of the 160 participants, not all responded to the demographic items.

percent of participants on varenicline (**Fig. 2**) reported nausea as the leading adverse effect experienced during treatment. The average creatinine level was 0.9 (SD = 0.2) for participants requiring creatinine evaluation.

The end-of-treatment cessation rate for both group and individual session participants was 64%, validated by a carbon monoxide reading of up to 8 ppm (**Fig. 3**). Follow-up telephone calls and/or e-mails revealed a self-report of tobacco abstinence of 12% at 3 months after treatment, 22% at 6 months, and 16% at 12 months. Eighty-two percent of participants (N = 130) at 12 months were lost to follow-up and were coded as tobacco dependent.

For participants receiving an individual session, the abstinence rates were lower than for the group session, with end-of-treatment abstinence rates of 55% compared with 66%. However, the follow-up abstinence rates were higher for the individual sessions than for the group sessions; outcomes at 3 months were 13% compared with 12%, at 6 months 26% compared with 21%, and at 12 months 17% compared with 16%.

Of 160 participants, 73 had Fagerström scores of 5 or more with the following cessation outcomes: 58.9% were tobacco free at the end of treatment followed by cessation rates of 9.6% at 3 months, 24.7% at 6 months, and 17.8% at 12 months. Similar trends were noted for CES-D scores. Thirty-nine participants had CES-D scores of 17 or more with the following cessation outcomes: 53.9% were tobacco free at the end of treatment followed by cessation rates of 15% at 3 months, 23.1% at 6 months, and 20.5% at 12 months. Participants who were non-GHSU affiliated (N = 13) had lower cessation rates, with 31% (N = 4) tobacco free at the end of treatment and 92% lost to follow-up and thus coded as relapsed with tobacco use. Only 1 non-GHSU participant reported a tobacco-free status for the follow-up telephone calls/e-mails at 3, 6, and 12 months.

| Table 2 Biological measures | | |
|---|---|---|
| Measure | Mean (SD) Baseline | Mean (SD) End of Treatment |
| Carbon monoxide | 19.2 (14.8) | 7.1 (10.4) |
| Systolic blood pressure | 130.1 (15.5) | 131.1 (17.7) |
| Diastolic blood pressure | 81.6 (11.0) | 82.1 (8.9) |
| Heart rate | 80.0 (14.1) | 78.4 (12.9) |
| Weight | 184.8 (45.3) | 188.5 (46.4) |

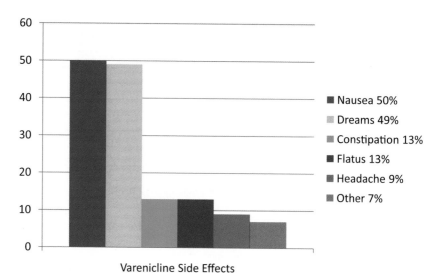

Varenicline Side Effects

**Fig. 2.** Medication profile.

Analysis by $\chi^2$ test revealed significant associations with abstinence rates at the end of treatment and at follow-up (3, 6, and 12 months) when compared with readiness-to-quit scores ($P = .0034$), number of sessions attended ($P = .0001$ for group and $P = .0342$ for individual), and if married ($P = .0312$). Participants not on pharmacotherapy had significant associations with lower quit rates at the end of treatment ($N = 15$; $P = .0001$) compared with those on pharmacotherapy.

## DISCUSSION

Although cessation rates decreased from 64% after end of treatment to 16% at 12 months, to the authors' knowledge, this is the first report of a nursing facility practice group dedicating resources for positive tobacco cessation outcomes in an academic

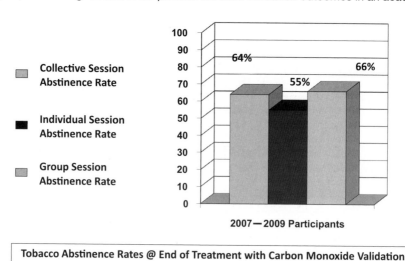

Tobacco Abstinence Rates @ End of Treatment with Carbon Monoxide Validation

**Fig. 3.** Abstinence rates: collective, group, and individual.

center–wide initiative. A meta-analysis of nursing interventions for smoking provides summary information on 14 studies involving nonhospitalized patients; 8 of these studies were considered high-intensity interventions. Compared with the authors' abstinence rate of 22% at 6 months, 3 of the 8 studies using high-intensity treatment had 6-month abstinence rates ranging between 14% and 17%. Compared with the authors' abstinence rates of 16% at 12 months, the other 5 studies reported 12-month quit rates between 2.6% and 7.9%.[16]

Similar to other studies, the association of abstinence rates at the end of treatment compared with nonpharmacotherapy use and pharmacotherapy for tobacco cessation treatment was significant.[13,17–19] Fifteen participants chose not to use pharmacotherapy, and, of those, only 4 were tobacco free at the end of treatment. A few characteristics about those who were successful compared with the others include lower Fagerström scores, lower CES-D scores, higher readiness-to-quit scores, and higher education. Although 27% were successful without medication at the end of treatment, at 6 months only 1 was tobacco free. This further supports the NFPG Tobacco Cessation Clinic's commitment to add to the body of knowledge for nurse-led, evidence-based, comprehensive approaches to promote long-term cessation success through pharmacotherapy and counseling.[16,20,21]

The amount of time dedicated to tobacco cessation treatment was a significant finding among the NFPG participants. The cessation rates for group counseling sessions (6 weeks, 2-hour sessions each week for a total of approximately 720 minutes) were consistent with the United States Public Health System guideline meta-analysis findings, which concluded that more intensive counseling (number of sessions/length of counseling) resulted in a higher cessation rate: 20.9% (odds ratio, 1.9; confidence interval, 1.6–2.2) at 6 months.[13] Similarly, the NFPG tobacco cessation program outcomes for individual counseling sessions (4 weeks, 1-hour sessions each week for a total of approximately 240 minutes) were consistent with a meta-analysis of 30 trials concluding that individual counseling was more effective than minimal/no counseling, with higher cessation rates at 6 months.[22] Whether participating in group or individual sessions, marital status was another significant finding. Similar to other studies, married NFPG participants had higher abstinence rates.[23,24]

Although the levels of nicotine dependence (Fagerström) and CES-D scores were not significantly associated with abstinence rates for the NFPG participants, there were clinically relevant observations. With an average Fagerström score of 4 (on a scale of 1 to 10), individuals with higher levels of nicotine dependence were noted to have lower cessation rates. This is consistent with research that has shown that a score of 6 or higher correlates with lower cessation rates.[25] The CES-D assessment for depression revealed an average score of 12 among the participants, and, similar to other reported studies, it was of clinical interest to note a higher rate of relapse associated with high CES-D scores (>17).[26] Future changes with the NFPG tobacco cessation protocol may include changing the CES-D cutoff from 20 to 17 and identifying participants at risk for relapse if the Fagerström score is 6 or higher.

All cessation end points consistently revealed lower abstinence rates at the 3-month follow-up compared with the 6-month and 12-month follow-up. This is consistent with the relapse literature and is believed to be associated with defensive cognitive restructuring.[27] Most participants were GHSU employees and students, therefore recognition of the NFPG Tobacco Cessation Clinic telephone number and e-mail was an easy way to avoid admitting a relapse. As time progressed, the telephone numbers and e-mails were not as recognizable, thus follow-up contact was established to confirm tobacco use status. Future changes for managing follow-up cessation data should include the gold standard of long-term cessation end points at 6 months and 12 months.[13]

Recognizing that positive tobacco cessation outcomes are well demonstrated with nurse-managed interventions[16,20,21]; the support of the GHSU leadership to cover the comprehensive treatment costs (medical evaluation, behavioral counseling, and pharmacotherapy) for a 2-year period during the Tobacco-Free Campus initiative was noteworthy. However, budgetary constraints limited the capacity to sustain end-of-treatment cessation rates through intensified follow-up and treatment. With the NFPG tobacco abstinence rate of 12% at 3 months and 22% at 6 months, funded initiatives for bolus treatment interventions and innovative follow-up strategies, such as text messaging, might have resulted in more term-positive long-term cessation outcomes.[28]

Opportunities abound with further evaluation of the effect of pharmacotherapy options among academic medical center employees and students. Considering that most participants received varenicline as the pharmacotherapy cessation aid of choice, the cessation outcomes and adverse medication effects of the NFPG Tobacco Cessation Clinic are consistent with the varenicline clinical trials.[17–19] Although the NFPG tobacco cessation outcomes cannot be generalized and most participants were lost to follow-up, the overall end-of-treatment abstinence rates support the use of first-line pharmacotherapy cessation aids approved by the US Food and Drug Administration, in combination with counseling, to significantly increase cessation rates.[13,16]

The main limitations of the NFPG tobacco cessation program are the lack of infrastructure support and resources to provide follow-up and expand capacity. The authors believe that this contributed to most participants being lost to follow-up and considered relapsed with their cessation attempt. During the time of the Tobacco-Free Policy initiative, GHSU did not have a robust electronic medical record system in place for tracking employees and students. Often e-mails went unopened and telephone messages were not returned. Funding did not support extensive follow-up with multiple mail-out correspondence, and a decision was made to limit follow-up attempts to 2 e-mails and 2 phone calls. Although the intent of the NFPG Tobacco Cessation Clinic was to become self-sustaining after the end of the 2-year plan for free treatment for GHSU employees and students, the interest in participation has declined. At present, enrollment has decreased by 75%, with an average cohort of 4 to 6 participants approximately 6 times per year.

## SUMMARY

Despite the decrease in tobacco use in the state of Georgia, the link between mortality and tobacco dependence remains too high to be ignored. It is well documented that nurses have been repeatedly associated with making a difference in the lives of tobacco-dependent individuals through effective tobacco cessation interventions. The experiences and outcomes of the GHSU NFPG Tobacco Cessation Clinic are encouraging for others to model. With cessation rates higher than national rates at the end of counseling session treatment, academic medical centers have an opportunity to evaluate the return on the investment for health among tobacco-dependent employees, students, and community members.

If progress is to be made toward ending the tobacco problem, nursing faculty practice plans must strategically prioritize and integrate tobacco cessation interventions with education, research, and advocacy. Only when tobacco cessation interventions are evidence based, interdisciplinary, and intense will a sustainable model of integrated practice be sustained. Nurse educators and researchers need to set outcome-driven research agendas targeting fundable venues that support proactive disease management treatment for tobacco-dependent individuals. Academic nurse leaders have a responsibility to drive practice outcomes to reduce tobacco-related morbidity and mortality rates and associated health care costs.

## ACKNOWLEDGMENTS

The authors acknowledge Dr Sharon Bennett for tireless hours of leadership and service with the NFPG Tobacco Cessation Clinic; Dr Dan Rahn, former GHSU President, for the Tobacco- Free Campus vision and leadership; Bryan Ginn, GHSU Assistant to the President for External Affairs, for championing for nurses with the Tobacco-Free Campus Initiative; Dr Lucy Marion, Dean GHSU College of Nursing, for reactivating the Nursing Faculty Practice Group; and Grover M. Hickson, III, RPh, and Kimbly Walker-Henley, PharmD, for the Kroger Pharmacy partnership and clinical support.

## REFERENCES

1. CDC. State specific prevalence of cigarette smoking and smokeless tobacco use among adults—United States 2009. MMWR Morb Mortal Wkly Rep 2010;59(43): 1401–6.
2. CDC. 2005 Georgia Youth Risk Behavior Survey. YRBSS online: comprehensive results. Interactive query system. 2005. Available at: http://apps.nccd.cdc.gov/youthonline/App/Results.aspx?LID=GA. Accessed August 15, 2011.
3. CDC. Smoking-attributable mortality, years of potential life lost, and productivity losses—United States, 2000–2004. MMWR Morb Mortal Wkly Rep 2008; 57(45):1226–8. Available at: http://www.cdc.gov/mmwr/preview/mmwrhtml/mm5745a3.htm. Accessed August 15, 2011.
4. Mokdak AH, Marks JS, Stroup DF, et al. Actual causes of death in the U.S. 2000. JAMA 2004;291(10):1238–41.
5. Georgia Health Sciences University News and Information. GHSU is tobacco-free. 2007. Available at: http://www.georgiahealth.edu/tobaccofree/. Accessed August 20, 2011.
6. Fichtenberg CM, Glantz SA. Effect of a smoke-free workplace on smoking behaviour: systematic review. BMJ 2002;325:188–95.
7. Georgia Health Sciences University School of Nursing. Nursing Faculty Practice Group. 2010. Available at: http://www.georgiahealth.edu/son/nfpg.htm. Accessed August 20, 2011.
8. Georgia Health Sciences University School of Nursing. Tobacco Cessation Clinic. 2010. Available at: http://www.georgiahealth.edu/son/tcc.htm. Accessed August 15, 2011.
9. Dracup K. Impact of faculty practice on an academic institution's mission and vision. Nurs Outlook 2004;52(4):174–8.
10. Sawyer MJ, Alexander IM, Gordon L, et al. A critical review of current nursing faculty practice. J Am Acad Nurse Pract 2000;12(12):511–6.
11. Saxe JM, Burgel BJ, Stringari-Murray S, et al. What is faculty practice? Nurs Outlook 2004;52(4):166–73.
12. Heath J, Andrews J. Using evidence-based educational strategies to increase knowledge and skills in tobacco cessation. Nurs Res 2006;55(Suppl 4):S44–50.
13. Fiore MC, Jaen CR, Baker TB, et al. Treating tobacco use and dependence: 2008 update. Clinical practice guideline. Public Health Service. Rockville (MD): US Department of Health and Human Services; 2008.

14. American Lung Association. Freedom from smoking 2011. Available at: http://www.lungusa.org/associations/states/florida/educational-programs/freedom-from-smoking/. Accessed August 20, 2011.
15. Nurses for Tobacco Control Coalition. The REAP framework (research, education, advocacy and practice) to advance tobacco control. Available at: http://www.nurses4tobaccocontrol.org/. Accessed August 15, 2011.
16. Gonzales D, Rennard SI, Nides M, et al. Varenicline, an α4β2 nicotinic acetylcholine receptor agonist, vs sustained-release bupropion and placebo for smoking cessation: randomized controlled trial. JAMA 2006;296(1):47–55.
17. Jorenby DE, Hays JT, Rogotti NA, et al. Efficacy of varenicline, an α4β2 nicotinic acetylcholine receptor partial agonist, vs placebo or sustained-release bupropion for smoking cessation: a randomized controlled trial. JAMA 2006;296(1):56–63.
18. Tonstad S, Tonnesen P, Hajek P, et al. Effect of maintenance therapy with varenicline on smoking cessation: a randomized controlled trial. JAMA 2006;296(1):64–71.
19. Rice VH, Stead LF. Nursing interventions for smoking cessation. Cochrane Database Syst Rev 2008;1:CD001188.
20. Ginn MB, Cox G, Heath J. An evidence-based approach to an in-patient tobacco cessation protocol. AACN Adv Crit Care 2008;19(3):268–78.
21. Heath J, Young S, Bennett S, et al. Evidence-based smoking cessation interventions for acute respiratory disorders. Annu Rev Nurs Res 2009;27:273–96.
22. Lancaster T, Stead LF. Individual behavioral counseling for smoking cessation. Cochrane Database Syst Rev 2008;4:CD001292.
23. Broms U, Silventoin K, Lahelma E, et al. Smoking cessation by socioeconomic status and marital status: the contribution of smoking behavior and family background. Nicotine Tob Res 2004;6(3):447–55.
24. Christakis NA, Fowler JH. The collective dynamics of smoking in a large social network. N Engl J Med 2008;358:2249–58.
25. Fagerstrom KO, Schneider NG. Measuring nicotine dependence: a review of the Fagerstrom Tolerance Questionnaire. J Behav Med 1989;12(2):159–82.
26. Paperwalla KN, Levin TT, Weiner J, et al. Smoking and depression. Nurs Clin North Am 2004;88(6):1483–94.
27. Piasecki TM. Relapse to smoking. Clin Psychol Rev 2006;26(2):196–215.
28. Free C, Knight R, Robertson S, et al. Smoking cessation support delivered via mobile phone text messaging (txt2stop): a single-blind, randomized trial. Lancet 2011;378:49–55.

# Prenatal Hair Nicotine Analysis in Homes with Multiple Smokers

Kristin Ashford, PhD, APRN, RN*, Susan Westneat, MA

KEYWORDS

- Pregnancy • Secondhand smoke • Biomarker • Preterm birth
- Nicotine

Primary smoking during pregnancy places a woman at greater risk for preterm delivery, preterm premature rupture of membranes, and delivering a low birth weight or small for gestational age infant.[1] Although there is less evidence regarding the effect of secondhand smoke (SHS) on perinatal morbidity, increased risk for decreased birth weight, smaller head circumference, stillbirth, and preterm birth have been consistently reported.[2–5]

SHS is defined as smoke inhaled by an individual who is not actively engaged in smoking but who is exposed to ambient tobacco smoke.[6] SHS consists of 2 components: sidestream smoke and mainstream smoke. Sidestream smoke refers to the smoke emitted from tobacco products, whereas mainstream smoke refers to the smoke exhaled by smokers. SHS contains approximately 4000 chemicals, causes nearly 3000 cases of lung cancer deaths among nonsmokers each year, and affects more than 22 million children in the United States annually.[7]

Biomarker validation is recommended to confirm smoking and SHS because of a high deception rate for self-report status caused by the social pressures attributed to smoking during pregnancy.[8] Whether a woman smokes during pregnancy or is exposed to SHS, biomarkers of exposure can be detected in both the mother and the infant.[9–11] Nicotine in maternal hair is a valid biomarker strongly associated with prenatal reports of SHS exposure.[12]

Funding: This study was funded by a University of Kentucky Faculty Research Grant and completed in part by a United States Public Health Service grant supporting the University of Kentucky General Clinical Research Center #M01RR02602. This publication was made possible by grant number K12DA14040 from the Office of Women's Health Research and the National Institute on Drug Abuse at the National Institute of Health. Its contents are solely the responsibility of the authors and do not necessarily represent the official views of National Institutes of Health.

University of Kentucky, College of Nursing, #417 College of Nursing Building, Lexington, KY 40536-0232, USA
* Corresponding author.
*E-mail address:* khashf0@uky.edu

Research examining the association between prenatal smoking, SHS exposure, and number of household smokers is limited. The purpose of the study was to examine the relationship between the levels of nicotine in maternal and infant hair and the number of household smokers among women who smoke and who are exposed to SHS during pregnancy. The aim of the study was to (1) examine the difference in maternal hair nicotine in smoking and SHS-exposed women in homes with 1, 2, or more additional smokers in the home; (2) examine the difference in infant hair nicotine in smoking and SHS-exposed women in homes with 1, 2, or more additional household smokers; and (3) describe the relationship between hair nicotine levels and preterm birth in homes with multiple smokers.

## METHODS
### Study Design and Population

A correlational, cross-sectional study design was used to determine the association between perinatal exposure to home SHS and nicotine levels in hair. Before data collection, the study was approved by the University of Kentucky Institutional Review Board, and all participants provided informed consent. Potential study participants were identified between December 2006 and April 2007 at the University Hospital. To be included in the study, women had to be at least 18 years of age, with singleton gestation, and have maternal scalp hair of at least 2 cm in length. Women were excluded if their pregnancy resulted in stillbirth, neonatal death, and/or delivery of an infant with severe congenital anomalies. Women with documented use of any drugs of abuse during pregnancy were also excluded. In the 4-month data collection period, there were 656 births, with nearly 85% meeting eligibility requirements. Quota sampling was used to ensure a representative distribution of mothers who were smokers, nonsmokers/SHS exposed, and nonsmokers/nonexposed during pregnancy.

A total of 210 women consented to participate within 3 days of their infant's birth. Mothers were identified via the Labor and Birth Daily Census Report and approached about participating while in the postpartum unit. After obtaining written consent, mothers were asked to complete a questionnaire. After collection of urine and hair samples by trained research assistants, participants were offered a choice of 2 incentives: a payment of $25 or the equivalent of $25 in diapers and wipes.

### Classification of Smoking and SHS Exposure

A woman was classified as a self-reported smoker if she responded "yes" to the question, "Have you smoked a cigarette, even a puff, in the past 7 days." Mothers who smoked were asked to classify their daily smoking consumption over the last 30 days as less than 1 cigarette, 1 to 5, 6 to 10, 11 to 15, 16 to 20, 21 to 25, 31 to 35, 36 to 40, and more than 40. Classification of SHS exposure was based on self-reports after confirmation of nonsmoking status. Nonsmokers were defined by a urine cotinine level of up to 99 ng/mL, and current smokers were defined by a urine cotinine level of 100 ng/mL or more. Previous reports on classification of smoking status using urine cotinine levels have yielded sensitivity and specificity of 88% and 92%, respectively.[13] Number of home SHS exposure sources was defined by the number of persons living in the participant's home (for >1 month) who smoked tobacco products. If the participant did not report any prenatal exposures to SHS in the home, vehicle, or workplace, they were classified as nonsmoking, nonexposed. If a participant answered "yes" or quantified exposure (hours or days) to any of the smoking exposure questions, they were classified as nonsmoking/SHS exposed.

## Collection of Maternal and Newborn Hair

Maternal hair samples were collected by cutting a proximal segment of hair (approximately 20–25 strands) from the posterior vertex nearest to the scalp and placed in a paper envelope. Collection of newborn hair involved cutting a pencil-width segment of hair behind the ear, placing it in a paper envelope, and storing it until the samples were mailed to Wellington Hospital, Wellington, New Zealand for analysis. Additional information regarding maternal and infant hair nicotine collection and analyses has been reported previously.[14]

## Statistical Analysis

With an effective sample size of 210 mothers and an $\alpha$ level of 0.05, the power of Spearman rank correlation to detect a significant association as small as 0.2 was calculated to be at least 80%. Univariate analyses were used to summarize the demographic and socioeconomic characteristics of the participants (**Table 1**). Age and number of smokers in the home are presented as mean values. The distribution of nicotine levels in hair was positively skewed, thus data were log transformed. Nicotine levels in hair are presented as geometric means and 95% confidence intervals. Data were analyzed using SAS version 9.3; an $\alpha$ level of 0.05 was used throughout.

## RESULTS

The demographics of the participants are given in **Table 1**. The mean age of the participants who smoked was 24.3 years compared with 24.8 years for those who were exposed to SHS. Fifty-three of the 210 participants were categorized as smokers and 157 as nonsmokers. Of the nonsmokers, 66 were classified as exposed to SHS, all of whom reported their home as the primary exposure site. Women who smoked during pregnancy had a mean of 2.4 additional smokers in the home compared with 1.2 for women who were exposed to SHS.

Maternal and infant hair samples were collected in nearly all the participants (99% of mothers, 98% of infants). There was no significant difference in demographics between mothers who smoked and those who were exposed to SHS, with the exception of college education. Significant differences in nicotine levels in maternal hair

**Table 1**
**Demographics and smoking classification (N = 210)**

| | Smoker n = 53 (%) | Nonsmoker/Passive n = 66 (%) | Nonsmoker/Nonexposed n = 91 (%) |
|---|---|---|---|
| Ethnicity/race | | | |
| White | 41 (19.5) | 33 (15.7) | 45 (21.4) |
| African American | 10 (4.8) | 14 (6.7) | 8 (3.8) |
| Hispanic | 0 | 18 (8.6) | 35 (16.7) |
| Marital status | | | |
| Single | 37 (17.7) | 40 (18.9) | 7 (13) |
| Married | 15 (7.2) | 26 (12.4) | 64 (30.6) |
| Highest grade completed | | | |
| Less than high school | 22 (11.1) | 13 (6.2) | 23 (11.0) |
| High school/GED | 17 (8.1) | 25 (12) | 20 (9.6) |
| Some college and above | 14 (6.7) | 27 (12.9) | 48 (23) |

existed between women exposed to SHS and women who smoked during pregnancy when comparing hair nicotine with 1, 2, or more smokers in the home (1 smoker at home, 0.0942 and 1.9279; 2 or more smokers at home, 0.1094 and 1.0501, respectively). Women who smoked during pregnancy had nearly twice the exposure time (hours) compared with women who were exposed to SHS (79.8 hours and 45 hours, respectively). See **Figs. 1** and **2** for the associations between household smoking and mean levels of maternal-infant hair nicotine.

Maternal hair significantly correlated with all smoking behaviors measured and had stronger association with smoking behavior than infant hair (**Table 2**). Infant hair demonstrated weaker but significant association in the reported smoking behaviors. Number of cigarettes smoked by other household members in the home ranged between 1 and 40 cigarettes per day, with a mean of 12.5 cigarettes per day. Half of the mothers who smoked during pregnancy reported smoking 1 to 10 cigarettes per day; 28% reported smoking 11 to 20 cigarettes per day; and 22% reported smoking more than 20 cigarettes per day. The total number of cigarettes smoked per day strongly correlated with nicotine levels in both maternal and infant hair.[14]

More than two-thirds of the preterm infants were born from women who smoked (36%) or who were exposed to SHS (33%) during pregnancy. Infants whose mother lived with 2 or more smokers in the home were nearly twice as likely to be transferred to the neonatal intensive care unit (NICU) compared with those with 1 smoker in the home. There were no significant differences in demographics regarding NICU admission when comparing women who smoked with women exposed to SHS.

## DISCUSSION

Levels of nicotine in maternal and infant hair increased as the number of smokers in the home increased. Evidence continues to stress the strong association between exposure to SHS and poor birth outcomes[5,15]; however, measurement of the number of household smokers is seldom reported and/or related with perinatal outcomes.

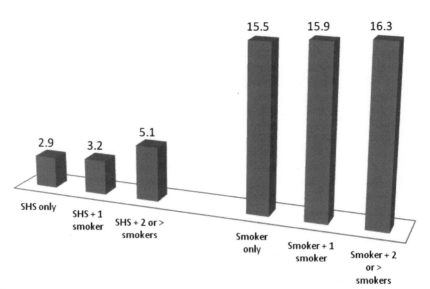

**Fig. 1.** Mean nicotine levels (ng/mL) for maternal hair (n = 201).

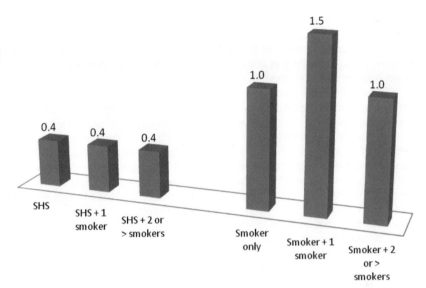

**Fig. 2.** Mean nicotine levels (ng/mL) for infant hair (n = 178).

Consistent with a previous report, this study demonstrates a significant association between the level of nicotine in maternal hair and the number of smokers in the home.[16] However, the association between the level of nicotine in infant hair and the number of smokers in the home was weaker than the association with maternal hair.

Other perinatal exposure considerations include dose-response relationships and hair nicotine reference values. Dose-response relationships between urine cotinine and home exposure in children and nonpregnant adults have been widely reported.[17,18] The dose-response relationship between the number of smokers in the home and perinatal outcomes is less clear. Fantuzzi and colleagues[16] (2007) recently noted a significant association between the number of home smokers and early preterm birth (<35 weeks' gestation). Previous examination of prenatal segmental hair nicotine analysis reported proximal mean concentrations in 3 smoking behavior classifications: nonsmoking, 2.8 ng/mL; exposed, 4.3 ng/mL; and active smoking, 11.08 ng/mL.[19] Similar trends in the nicotine concentrations (ng/mL) of maternal hair segments were noted in our study (0.33, 1.02, and 9.6, respectively). Hair sampling

**Table 2**
Spearman rank correlations among hair nicotine and smoking variables (*P*<.05)

| Self-Reported Smoking Variables | Hair Nicotine Level | |
| --- | --- | --- |
| | Maternal Hair | Infant Hair |
| Smoking status | 0.74 | 0.39 |
| Number of cigarettes per day | 0.68 | 0.45 |
| Total SHS exposure[a] | 0.68 | 0.28 |
| Two or more adults smoking in home | 0.61 | 0.23 |

[a] Total SHS exposure accounts for home, workplace, and vehicle.

size may account for the lower nicotine concentrations in the present study. In both studies, maternal hair nicotine (unlike infant hair) was able to significantly differentiate between the 3 smoking classifications. Prenatal mean hair nicotine concentrations range from 1.5 to 1.9 ng/mg in active smokers and 0.04 to 0.09 ng/mg in passively exposed women; however, the recommended cutoff value for prenatal hair cotinine level to distinguish active smokers from passive smokers is 0.2 ng/mL.[20]

During pregnancy and postpartum, a woman's primary location for exposure to SHS is in her home; the primary exposure source is her spouse and/or significant other.[21] In this study, her significant other was most often defined as spouse, partner, and/or infant's father, followed by mother or mother-in-law. Home smoking restrictions or home smoking bans/policies can decrease and/or prolong relapse rates in pregnant and/or postpartum women.[21–24] Conversely, homes where smoking is allowed have higher prenatal smoking rates.[25] Having home smoking restrictions has also been reported to influence intentions to quit smoking.[26] Although sustained smoking cessation provides the most benefits for decreasing perinatal exposure to SHS, consideration for a reduction of smoke could offer health benefits to the family.[24] Few studies have evaluated the relationship between a maternal home smoking ban and perinatal outcomes. Yoo and colleagues[27] (2010) concluded that spouses' who smoked outside the home did not reduce overall exposure to pregnant women compared with nonsmoking spouses.

Limitations in the present study exist and should be addressed. First, self-reports of smoking and exposure to SHS during pregnancy can result in high deception rates; however, only 3% of confirmed smokers via urine cotinine reported nonsmoking status. Second, all participants were recruited from a local hospital, which may limit generalizability. Third, sampling error cannot be calculated with quota sampling methods. Fourth, ethnic hair nicotine differences were not accounted for because of sample size and statistical limitations. In the present study, ethnicity would have greatly reduced group sizes when examining SHS and smoking behaviors in homes with 1, 2, or more smokers in the home. Finally, measurement of nicotine in maternal and infant hair was performed at one time point. Although, nicotine in hair is a very stable marker of long-term exposure, collection during each trimester would offer a more comprehensive and valid assessment regarding smoking and exposure status.

Strengths in the study include biochemical validation of the smoking status of pregnant women; use of nicotine in hair as a valid and long-term biomarker of exposure to SHS; collection of both maternal and infant hair samples; and collection of several self-reported measures of exposure to SHS at home (hours per day, number of exposure sources, and number of household smokers).

## SUMMARY

Maternal hair is a more valid and sensitive measure of number of household smokers than infant hair. Pregnant women who smoke or who are exposed to SHS are more likely to experience a multitude of adverse perinatal outcomes than those who do not smoke and/or are not exposed. Furthermore, pregnant women living in households with 2 or more smokers are more likely to have their infant admitted to the NICU immediately after birth. Health care providers and clinical nurse leaders are strongly encouraged to educate all clients about the adverse perinatal effects of smoking and SHS exposure among pregnant women. Compromised infants face a multitude of acute and lifelong health issues; thus, a significant percentage of adverse outcomes could be prevented by avoiding primary and secondary smoking during pregnancy. Prevention strategies including home smoking bans and focused public media campaigns on the harmful effects of SHS exposure are necessary to avoid the adverse perinatal outcomes associated with SHS.

## REFERENCES

1. US Department of Health and Human Services, Public Health Service. Women and smoking: a report of the Surgeon General. Washington, DC: Office of the Surgeon General; 2001.
2. Ashford KB, Hahn E, Hall L, et al. The effects of prenatal secondhand smoke exposure on preterm birth and neonatal outcomes. J Obstet Gynecol Neonatal Nurs 2010;39(5):525–35.
3. Hegaard HK, Kjaergaard H, Moller LF, et al. The effect of environmental tobacco smoke during pregnancy on birth weight. Acta Obstet Gynecol Scand 2006; 85(6):675–81.
4. CDC. The health consequences of involuntary exposure to tobacco smoke: a report of the Surgeon General. Atlanta (GA): Department of Health and Human Services, Public Health Service, Centers for Disease Control and Prevention, National Center for Chronic Disease and Prevention and Promotion, Office of Smoking and Health; 2006.
5. Salmasi G, Grady R, Jones J, et al. Environmental tobacco smoke exposure and perinatal outcomes: a systematic review and meta-analyses. Acta Obstet Gynecol Scand 2010;89(4):423–41.
6. Klerman L. Protecting children: reducing their environmental tobacco smoke exposure. Nicotine Tob Res 2004;6(Suppl 2):S239–53.
7. US Department of Health and Human Services. Involuntary exposure to tobacco smoke: a report of the Surgeon General. Atlanta (GA): US Department of Health and Human Services, Centers for Disease Control and Prevention, National Center on Chronic Disease Prevention and Health Promotion, Office on Smoking and Health; 2006.
8. Webb DA, Boyd NR, Messina D, et al. The discrepancy between self-reported smoking status and urine cotinine levels among women enrolled in prenatal care at four publicly funded clinical sites. J Public Health Manag Pract 2003; 9(4):322–5.
9. Klein J, Blanchette P, Koren G. Assessing nicotine metabolism in pregnancy– a novel approach using hair analysis. Forensic Sci Int 2004;145(2–3):191–4.
10. Eliopoulos C, Klein J, Phan MK, et al. Hair concentrations of nicotine and cotinine in women and their newborn infants. JAMA 1994;271(8):621–3.
11. Jacqz-Aigrain E, Zhang ED, Maillard G, et al. Maternal smoking during pregnancy and nicotine and cotinine concentrations in maternal and neonatal hair. BJOG 2002;109(8):909–11.
12. Sorensen M, Bisgaard H, Stage M, et al. Biomarkers of exposure to environmental tobacco smoke in infants. Biomarkers 2007;12(1):38–46.
13. Bernert JT, Harmon TL, Sosnoff CS, et al. Technical note: use of cotinine immunoassay test strips for preclassifying urine samples from smokers and nonsmokers prior to analysis by LCMSMS. J Anal Toxicol 2005;29:814–8.
14. Ashford KB, Hahn E, Hall L, et al. Measuring prenatal secondhand smoke exposure in mother–baby couplets. Nicotine Tob Res 2010;12(2):127–35.
15. Khader Y, Al-Akour N, AlZubi I, et al. The association between second hand smoke and low birth weight and preterm delivery. Matern Child Health J 2011; 15(4):453–9.

16. Fantuzzi G, Aggazzotti G, Righi E, et al. Preterm delivery and exposure to active and passive smoking during pregnancy: a case–control study from Italy. Paediatr Perinat Epidemiol 2007;21(3):194–200.

17. Yousey YK. Household characteristics, smoking bans, and passive smoke exposure in young children. J Pediatr Health Care 2006;20(2):98–105.

18. Al-Delaimy WK, Crane J, Woodward A. Is the hair nicotine level a more accurate biomarker of environmental tobacco smoke exposure than urine cotinine? J Epidemiol Community Health 2002;56(1):66–71.

19. Pichini S, Garcia-Algar O, Munoz L, et al. Assessment of chronic exposure to cigarette smoke and its change during pregnancy by segmental analysis of maternal hair nicotine. J Expo Anal Environ Epidemiol 2003;13(2):144.

20. Florescu A, Ferrence R, Einarson TR, et al. Reference values for hair cotinine as a biomarker of active and passive smoking in women of reproductive age, pregnant women, children, and neonates: systematic review and meta-analysis. Ther Drug Monit 2007;29(4):437–46.

21. Sockrider MM, Hudmon KS, Addy R, et al. An exploratory study of control of smoking in the home to reduce infant exposure to environmental tobacco smoke. Nicotine Tob Res 2003;5(6):901–10.

22. Yunsheng M, Goins KV, Pbert L, et al. Predictors of smoking cessation in pregnancy and maintenance postpartum in low-income women. Matern Child Health J 2005;9(4):393–402.

23. McBride CM, Curry SJ, Lando HA, et al. Prevention of relapse in women who quit smoking during pregnancy. Am J Public Health 1999;89(5):706–11.

24. Severson HH, Andrews JA, Lichtenstein E, et al. Reducing maternal smoking and relapse: long-term evaluation of a pediatric intervention. Prev Med 1997;26(1):120–30.

25. Orr ST, Newton E, Tarwater PM, et al. Factors associated with prenatal smoking among black women in eastern North Carolina. Matern Child Health J 2005;9(3):245–52.

26. Gilpin EA, White MM, Farkas AJ, et al. Home smoking restrictions: which smokers have them and how they are associated with smoking behavior. Nicotine Tob Res 1999;1(2):153–62.

27. Yoo SH, Paek YJ, Kim SS, et al. Hair nicotine levels in non-smoking pregnant women whose spouses smoke outside of the home. Tob Control 2010;19(4):318–24.

# Evidence-Based Smoking Cessation for College Students

Karen M. Butler, DNP, RN[a],*, Amanda Fallin, PhD, RN[b],
S. Lee Ridner, PhD, APRN[c]

## KEYWORDS

- College students • Smoking prevention and cessation
- Smoke-free policy

Despite years of prevention and control efforts on US college campuses, tobacco use remains a problem among college students. Recent national data reveal that after alcohol, the next most commonly used substance is tobacco. According to the American College Health Association (ACHA)-National College Health Assessment[1] conducted in the fall of 2010, 85% of college students described themselves as nonsmokers (never smoked or have not smoked cigarettes in the last 30 days). The purpose of this article is to give an overview of what is known about cigarette smoking among college students, present existing evidence-based interventions for smoking prevention, cessation, and exposure to secondhand smoke (SHS) on college campuses, and make recommendations for future research.

## OVERVIEW OF THE PROBLEM

Cigarette smoking is the leading cause of preventable morbidity and mortality in the United States, contributing to nearly 440,000 deaths annually. In addition, there is no safe level of exposure to SHS; exposure has immediate adverse health effects.[2] The ACHA[3] recognizes the health risks of tobacco use and exposure to SHS and has therefore adopted a No Tobacco Use policy, encouraging colleges and universities to work to achieve a 100% indoor and outdoor campus-wide tobacco-free environment. The ACHA also actively supports the Healthy Campus 2020 goals to increase the percentage of students who receive information on tobacco use

[a] Tobacco Policy Research Program, College of Nursing, University of Kentucky, 423 College of Nursing Building, Lexington, KY 40536, USA
[b] Center for Tobacco Control Research and Education, University of California, San Francisco, 530 Parnassus Avenue, San Francisco, CA 94143, USA
[c] School of Nursing, University of Louisville, 555 South Floyd Street, Louisville, KY 40292, USA
* Corresponding author.
E-mail address: Karen.Butler@uky.edu

Nurs Clin N Am 47 (2012) 21–30
doi:10.1016/j.cnur.2011.10.007
0029-6465/12/$ – see front matter © 2012 Elsevier Inc. All rights reserved.

prevention, reduce the percentage of college students who smoke cigarettes, and increase student participation in smoke-free campus initiatives.

Nationally, adults aged 18–24 years (the age range for traditional college students) have the highest prevalence of smoking at 23.7%.[4] After peaking at about 30% in the past decade,[5,6] the current reported smoking prevalence among college students is 14.9%.[7] Of students who are current smokers (reported use within the past 30 days), 1 in 3 smokes everyday. The same report indicates that college students believe tobacco use to be more common among their peers than it actually is. Students perceived that 82.7% of their peers were current smokers and that only 17.3% were nonsmokers, indicating that many students view smoking as a normal, common occurrence among their peers.

Most college student smokers began smoking in high school, having started by the 12th grade and continuing into college. Men and women have similar smoking rates, with men having slightly higher rates than women (20.9% vs 18.1%).[8] College students who smoke are more likely to be Caucasian and least likely to be African American.[9] College students who drink alcohol are more likely to initiate smoking.[10,11] Tobacco and alcohol are more likely to be used concurrently among this group, which may also facilitate tobacco use. Wechsler and colleagues[12(p1693)] found that among college smokers, 11% had their first cigarette and 28% began to smoke regularly at or after the age of 18. Concurrent use of alcohol and tobacco is highly correlated in both clinical and nonclinical samples of college students. Data from a national survey indicated that 98% of college smokers drink alcohol, and 44% to 59% of college student drinkers also smoke cigarettes.[13]

Approximately half of all college smokers may be social smokers,[14] and most use unique criteria to identify themselves. Berg and colleagues[15] identified how college students define the term "smoker" and how this definition impacts smoking behavior and attitudes. A smoker was described in terms of smoking frequency, contextual factors (ie, smoking alone vs smoking at parties, time since initiation of smoking, purchasing vs borrowing cigarettes, and level of addiction [can one quit without great effort]), and whether smoking is a habit. Using such criteria to define oneself as a smoker or nonsmoker influences both motivation to and perception of the need to quit.

Other researchers found that more than half of the students (56.3%) denied being smokers in spite of their current smoking behavior.[16] Most of these smokers referred to themselves as social smokers. This group was likely to smoke infrequently, say they were not addicted to cigarettes, have mostly nonsmokers as close friends, prefer dating nonsmokers, and smoke for reasons other than stress relief. Walker and colleagues[17] had similar findings in that college students who self-identified as nonsmokers reported smoking and discussed their smoking behaviors in the context of smoking while stressed, while drinking, and when with friends. Moran and colleagues[14] found social smoking to be a distinct pattern of tobacco use common among college students, which may represent a stage in the uptake of smoking. College students who identify themselves as social smokers generally believe that they will only smoke for a while; in other words, that they will not continue to smoke when they are no longer in the college environment.[18] In a study of smoking identity and smoking behaviors, Ridner and colleagues[19] found that students who self-identified as occasional and social smokers did not differ on the number of days they smoked, but 20% of current smokers identified themselves as nonsmokers. Recent research found that self-identified young adult social smokers may be a high-risk group with unique challenges for cessation and may be less likely to quit smoking.[20]

College students report smoking as a means of controlling stress or depression[9] and may use smoking as a means to let others know when they are distressed or unhappy.[21] Some college student groups have been found to have higher smoking rates than others. Smoking prevalence is higher among active members of fraternities and sororities than among students who are not members.[22] Smoking among college students is also linked to other risky behaviors. Researchers report that college student smokers are more likely to use alcohol and other substances and report experimenting with and using more than one other substance, such as alcohol, marijuana, cocaine, or other drugs, while smoking.[9] College smokers are more likely than nonsmokers to engage in high-risk alcohol use, risky driving, relational abuse, depression, less exercise, and use of emergency and mental health services.[23] In a college student sample, cigarette use, even at low levels, was associated with increased binge drinking and illicit substance use.[24]

Many college students are making attempts to quit smoking. A large national study found that half of the current college student smokers surveyed (N = 2014) tried to quit in the previous year. More striking was the finding that 18% had made 5 or more attempts to quit.[12] Smoking prevention and cessation programs have been implemented at many colleges and universities, but students continue to smoke. Existing tobacco cessation efforts run the gamut from individual and group counseling to campus-wide programs to policy initiatives such as smoke-free campuses and community smoke-free laws.

## STRATEGIES FOR PREVENTION AND CESSATION

The ACHA[3] took a strong position in 2009, recommending that all college campuses be tobacco free. The ACHA supports intervention at individual student, campus, and environmental levels to reduce tobacco use. Examples include cessation counseling (individual level), population-based programming (campus level), and banning tobacco use and advertising on campuses (environmental level).

### Individual and Campus Strategies

Smoking cessation interventions should focus on education, motivation, and behavior change, as these interventions have been shown to be effective. Smoking cessation counseling can be conducted in person (individual or group sessions) or over the telephone.[25] Telephone-based counseling can be either proactive or reactive. Proactive counseling involves making a series of calls to interested participants,[26] whereas reactive counseling involves providing cessation information on request. Even brief counseling interventions by health care providers have been shown to effectively promote smoking cessation.[27]

Other types of smoking cessation interventions use technology and are Internet or text message based.[28,29] RealU, an Internet-based smoking cessation program, was tested at the University of Minnesota. Participants received an online magazine with 4 articles tailored for college students; 1 of the 4 articles focused on smoking. The participants also received a weekly supportive e-mail from a peer. The program was structured around college life, so there was a break in the intervention scheduled during academic holidays and the week of final examinations. At the end of the intervention, the treatment group more frequently reported not smoking in the preceding 30 days than did the control group.[28]

Riley and colleagues[29] tested text message and online cessation programs at a large university in the Washington, DC, area. Text messages were tailored for participants based on the transtheoretical model as well as times of the day that a participant indicated he or she was most likely to be tempted to smoke. An example of a text message included "While studying, keep snacks such as pretzels, carrot sticks, etc., around."[(p246)] Participants could also text for assistance when they needed help with cravings to smoke. Six weeks after starting the program, 45% of the participants reported abstinence with 42% of the abstainers verified with cotinine levels. Participants who continued to smoke reported significantly reduced smoking rates and dependence. Overall, participants accepted the text messages.[29] These results show that such interventions may be effective, at least in the short-term, and can easily be implemented within the college student population.

A recent systematic review looking at mobile telephone–based interventions for smoking cessation found that short-term effects were positive, but there was no evidence of long-term effects.[30] Results showed that text message mobile telephone programs were effective in the short-term (6 weeks), and a combined Internet-mobile telephone program was effective for up to 12 months. More research is needed to identify strategies to promote the sustainability of these effects and determine whether such interventions can really help smokers quit in the long-term.

Contests are another potential strategy to encourage smoking cessation among college students. Rooney and colleagues[31] held Quit and Win contests with 152 participants at 3 postsecondary institutions in Wisconsin. Participants who successfully stopped smoking were eligible for a raffle for large gifts (eg, $1500 for travel) as well as small incentives (eg, free pizza). At the conclusion of the event, 30% of the participants reported that they had stopped smoking; 6 months later, the quit rate was 12%. The vast majority (94%) of participants responded positively about the potential for contests to help students stop smoking.

Recruitment and retention are important aspects of any smoking cessation program. Researchers have investigated factors associated with retention of college students in smoking cessation programs.[32,33] Factors associated with program attendance primarily include location and price. In a study of 193 college student smokers, 50% reported biking or walking as their primary means of transportation, and the majority preferred a location within 3 miles. Cost is also a factor in students' willingness to attend smoking cessation interventions.[32] The ACHA recommends offering non-cost-prohibitive smoking cessation interventions, including medications, for all college student smokers.

Davidson and colleagues[33] described strategies to recruit and retain college fraternity and sorority members who were current smokers into a cessation study. To enhance recruitment, researchers began relationship building with members of each fraternity and sorority chapter before initiation of the study, conducted raffles, and screened for study admission during existing chapter meetings. Of the eligible members, 76% agreed to participate. Other steps were taken to increase retention, such as the use of cash incentives, flexible scheduling, multiple reminders, chapter incentives, and use of chapter members as study personnel. The investigators believe that these strategies using partnership, convenience, and flexibility may be effective in engaging and recruiting similar samples to participate in smoking cessation studies.

## Environmental Strategies

Nationwide, the adoption of smoke-free policies in postsecondary institutions is a growing trend. As of July 2011, more than 500 college and university campuses had comprehensive smoke-free policies.[34] Results of several studies indicate that voluntary smoke-free policies have been associated with a reduction in smoking rates.[35] The North Carolina Tobacco-Free Colleges Initiative is an example of an initiative to encourage tobacco-free college campuses.[36] As part of the project, health departments or groups at the institution received grants to encourage policy development, compliance, and smoking cessation. Groups moved toward these goals by building coalitions to promote policy adoption. Groups also reached out to specific at-risk populations such as college freshmen. After 5 years, the number of tobacco-free colleges in North Carolina increased from 1 to 33. Diffusion of these policies was faster among colleges involved in the project.

College students support smoke-free policies.[37–39] In a national survey of approximately 11,000 students at 119 postsecondary institutions, approximately 75% responded that they supported smoke-free buildings and dining and residence halls.[38] Among a sample of 2260, college students voiced some support for smoke-free campus policies because they provide protection for nonsmokers from SHS and lead to less cigarette litter.[37] Thompson and colleagues[39] surveyed more than 14,000 postsecondary students in Washington, Oregon, and Idaho and found that approximately 82% of the students responded that clean air was more important than the ability to smoke.

Tobacco advertisements on college and university campuses are another relevant environmental issue. College students are heavily targeted by the tobacco industry as potential young customers.[40] Promotions are held in bars and other venues to encourage smoking as a social norm, moving them from social to regular (pack a day) smoking. College students are significant to the tobacco industry because they are in a stage of transition from adolescence to adulthood, which makes them particularly vulnerable to developing lifelong nicotine dependence. The tobacco industry spent more than $1 million a day in 2005 sponsoring events and giveaways targeting college students.[41] During the first 6 months of the 2000 to 2001 school year, almost 10% of the US college students surveyed reported attending a social event sponsored by the tobacco industry in which free cigarettes were distributed. College students at 115 of the 119 schools participating in the survey reported seeing tobacco promotions at a bar or nightclub; tobacco promotional events had occurred at 118 of these schools. Students' participation in these tobacco industry events was significantly associated with tobacco use.[41] In the national survey of college students by Rigotti and colleagues,[38] 71% favored a ban on tobacco industry sponsorship and advertisement on college campuses.

## Symptom Management

Smokers who make quit attempts are more likely to be successful if their symptoms are well managed. A large body of evidence supports using pharmacotherapies to control withdrawal symptoms during smoking cessation.[27] Options for first-line therapy include numerous forms of nicotine replacement, several classes of antidepressants, and nicotinic receptor agonists. The use of nicotine replacement therapy increases the likelihood of cessation from 50% to 70%.[42] Data also support the use of antidepressants and nicotinic receptor agonists for long-term cessation.[43,44]

There is little evidence to support medication use among light smokers (eg, those who smoke less than 10 cigarettes per day). In a study of African American light smokers, Ahluwalia and colleagues[45] found that nicotine replacement therapy did not improve cessation rates. Recent data from the ACHA show that only 1 in 3 college smokers do not smoke on a daily basis.[46] Of daily smokers on college campuses, 50% are classified as light smokers.[47] Because of the limited number of studies specifically examining light smokers, there is no clear guideline for the use of smoking cessation medications in this group. Fiore and colleagues[27] recommend that smaller doses be considered if nicotine replacement medications are prescribed for this group. There are no recommendations for using antidepressants or nicotinic receptor agonists for light smokers.

Among adult smokers, 70% want to quit smoking and 40% attempt to do so every year; unfortunately, only 5% succeed.[48] In a study of college smokers, Ridner and Hahn[49] found that 86% of the participants had made a serious attempt to quit smoking and an overwhelming majority (88%) had attempted to quit without any assistance. Unassisted quit attempts have the lowest chance of success when compared with other methods.[27] Therefore, it is important to provide a menu of options, including self-help materials, individual counseling, cessation groups, campus-wide programs, environmental strategies, and pharmacotherapy, to help college smokers succeed with cessation.

### Relapse Prevention

Relapse after smoking cessation is a significant problem; few smokers successfully achieve abstinence with quit attempts.[48] For college students, relapse typically occurs in social situations, in settings such as bars, or on returning to campus after a break. However, because there are multiple definitions of smoking abstinence (24 hours, 7 days, 6 months, or years) and not every lapse in smoking cessation results in relapse, assessment of college student relapse is difficult.[50,51] Because there is no clear-cut definition of abstinence, it is difficult to discern where smoking cessation treatment ends and relapse prevention begins.

Relapse prevention routinely involves interventions designed to boost the effects of smoking cessation interventions. Boosters can be in the form of cognitive and behavioral interventions that focus on identifying high-risk situations and developing skills to manage these situations or pharmacologic agents to aid in continued cessation. Several systematic reviews and meta-analyses of relapse prevention have provided mixed results.[51–53] Therefore, there is no clear evidence that relapse prevention is effective.

### College Health Care Providers

College health care providers are in an ideal position to take the lead on college campuses in providing multifaceted programming, which can positively impact smoking behaviors among college students. Every student should be screened for smoking every time he or she is seen by a college health care provider. However, despite the evidence that brief interventions by health care providers can impact smoking cessation, between one-third and one-fourth of college students seen by college health care providers report that they are not asked about smoking.[23,27,54] Of the students identified as smokers, 57% were advised to quit smoking and only 22% received specific advice on how to quit.[54] Lawrance and Lawler[55] found that only 20% of the college health care providers surveyed asked all or nearly all of their patients about smoking. Once smokers were identified, more than 95% of the providers reported advising patients to quit smoking. Several factors may influence the suboptimal interventions that college students receive.

In a study of college health care providers, Fagan[56] found that most providers thought that patients were resistant to advice on smoking cessation, there was a lack of resources to follow up cessation attempts, and acute care was a priority. The lack of training in smoking cessation counseling techniques may influence the care that college students receive.[23,56] Also, there is the perception among students and college health care providers that cessation services would not be used if available.[23,57] Halperin and colleagues[23] found that 60% of the students said they would not seek assistance but 20% of those, when prompted, stated they would use nicotine replacement if it were free. Unfortunately, college health care providers recommend nicotine replacement less than one-half the time for patients interested in cessation.[55]

In addition to the individual college health provider practices, the lack of formal cessation programs may be a barrier for college smokers. A national study of college health center directors found that more than 40% of the schools did not offer smoking cessation services.[57] A separate study with key informants from 50 US universities found that 44% did offer cessation programs but only 20% covered the costs of cessation medications,[23] despite the ACHA[3] recommendation that all universities offer cessation services, including medications, for free or at reduced costs.

## SUMMARY AND RECOMMENDATIONS FOR THE FUTURE

This article provides an overview of what is known about cigarette smoking among college students as well as existing interventions for smoking prevention, cessation, and exposure to SHS. Despite a strong stance by the ACHA and prevention and control efforts on US college campuses, smoking and exposure to SHS remain a problem among this population. Strategies to reduce tobacco use on college campuses have been identified, with many demonstrated to be effective, at least in the short-term. However, most strategies have not been proven to impact long-term abstinence in this population. Future research should build on what is known in order to design and test innovative, comprehensive interventions, including individual, campus-wide, community, and environmental strategies, with the goal of creating sustainable reductions in smoking behaviors among college students.

## REFERENCES

1. American College Health Association. American College Health Association-National College Health Assessment II: reference group data report fall 2010. Linthicum (MD): American College Health Association; 2011.
2. U.S. Department of Health and Human Services. The health consequences of smoking: a report of the Surgeon General. Atlanta (GA): U.S. Department of Health and Human Services, Centers for Disease Control and Prevention, National Center for Chronic Disease Prevention and Health Promotion, Office on Smoking and Health; 2004.
3. American College Health Association. ACHA guidelines: position statement on tobacco on college and university campuses. Hanover (MD): American College Health Association; 2009.
4. Centers for Disease Control and Prevention. Cigarette smoking among adults and trends in smoking cessation—United States, 2008. MMWR Morb Mortal Wkly Rep 2009;58(44):1227–32.
5. Johnston LD, O'Malley PM, Bachman JG. Monitoring the Future national survey results on adolescent drug use: overview of key findings, 2001. NIH Publication No. 02-5105. Bethesda (MD): National Institute on Drug Abuse; 2002. p. 56.
6. McKee SA, Hinson R, Rounsaville D, et al. Survey of subjective effects of smoking while drinking among college students. Nicotine Tob Res 2004;6(1):111–7.
7. American College Health Association. American College Health Association-National College Health Assessment spring 2007 reference group data report (abridged). J Am Coll Health 2008;56(5):469–79.
8. Johnston LD, O'Malley PM, Bachman JG. Monitoring the Future national survey results on drug use, 1975–2001. Volume II: college students and adults ages 19–40. NIH Publication No. 02-5107. Bethesda (MD): National Institute on Drug Abuse; 2002. p. 242.

9. Patterson F, Lerman C, Kaufmann VG, et al. Cigarette smoking practices among American college students: review and future directions. J Am Coll Health 2004; 52(5):203–10.
10. Staten RR, Noland M, Rayens MK, et al. Social influences on cigarette initiation among college students. Am J Health Behav 2007;31(4):353–62.
11. Wechsler H, Lee JE, Kuo M, et al. Trends in college binge drinking during a period of increased prevention efforts. Findings from 4 Harvard School of Public Health College Alcohol Study surveys: 1993-2001 [corrected] [Erratum appears in J Am Coll Health 2002;51(1):37]. J Am Coll Health 2002;50(5):203–17.
12. Wechsler H, Rigotti NA, Gledhill-Hoyt J, et al. Increased levels of cigarette use among college students: a cause for national concern. JAMA 1998;280(19): 1673–8.
13. Wechsler H, Lee JE, Nelson TF, et al. Underage college students' drinking behavior, access to alcohol, and the influence of deterrence policies. Findings from the Harvard School of Public Health College Alcohol Study. J Am Coll Health 2002;50(5):223–36.
14. Moran S, Wechsler H, Rigotti NA. Social smoking among US college students. Pediatrics 2004;114(4 Pt 1):1028–34.
15. Berg C, Parelkar P, Lessard L, et al. Defining "smoker": college student attitudes and related smoking characteristics. Nicotine Tob Res 2010;12:963–9.
16. Levinson AH, Campo S, Gascoigne J, et al. Smoking, but not smokers: identity among college students who smoke cigarettes. Nicotine Tob Res 2007;9(8): 845–52.
17. Walker KL, Ridner S, Hahn EJ. Exploratory study of young adults' perceptions of tobacco use and tobacco marketing. Int J Intercult Commun Stud 2007;16: 7–13.
18. Majchrzak N, Park E, Rigotti N. Tobacco use by Massachusetts college students: a qualitative study. Presented at the Annual Meeting, Society for Research in Nicotine and Tobacco. Savannah (GA), February, 2002.
19. Ridner SL, Walker KL, Hart JL, et al. Smoking identities and behavior: evidence of discrepancies, issues for measurement and intervention. West J Nurs Res 2010; 32(4):434–46.
20. Song AV, Ling PM. Social smoking among young adults: investigation of intentions and attempts to quit. Am J Public Health 2011;101(7):1291–6.
21. Nichter M, Nichter M, Carkoglu A, Tobacco Etiology Research Network. Reconsidering stress and smoking: a qualitative study among college students. Tob Control 2007;16(3):211–4.
22. McCabe SE, Schulenberg JE, Johnston LD, et al. Selection and socialization effects of fraternities and sororities on US college student substance use: a multi-cohort national longitudinal study. Addiction 2005;100(4):512–24.
23. Halperin AC, Smith SS, Heiligenstein E, et al. Cigarette smoking and associated health risks among students at five universities. Nicotine Tob Res 2009;12(2): 96–104.
24. Schorling JB, Gutgesell M, Klas P, et al. Tobacco, alcohol and other drug use among college students. J Subst Abuse 1994;6(1):105–15.
25. Chandler MA, Rennard SI. Smoking cessation. Chest 2010;137(2):428–35.
26. Coleman T, McEwen A, Bauld L, et al. Protocol for the proactive or reactive telephone smoking cessation support (PORTSSS) trial. Trials 2009;10(1):26.
27. Fiore M, Jaén C, Baker T, et al. Treating tobacco use and dependence: 2008 update. Clinical practice guideline. Rockville (MD): U.S. Department of Health and Human Services, Public Health Service; 2008.

28. An LC, Klatt C, Perry CL, et al. The RealU online cessation intervention for college smokers: a randomized controlled trial. Prev Med 2008;47(2):194–9.
29. Riley W, Obermayer J, Jean-Mary J. Internet and mobile phone text messaging intervention for college smokers. J Am Coll Health 2008;57(2):245–8.
30. Whittaker R, Borland R, Bullen C, et al. Mobile phone-based interventions for smoking cessation. Cochrane Database Syst Rev 2009;4:CD006611.
31. Rooney BL, Silha P, Gloyd J, et al. Quit and Win smoking cessation contest for Wisconsin college students. WMJ 2005;104(4):45–9.
32. Black DR, Loftus EA, Chatterjee R, et al. Smoking cessation interventions for university students: recruitment and program design considerations based on social marketing theory. Prev Med 1993;22(3):388–99.
33. Davidson MM, Cronk NJ, Harris KJ, et al. Strategies to recruit and retain college smokers in cessation trials. Res Nurs Health 2010;33(2):144–55.
34. Americans for Nonsmokers' Rights. U.S. colleges and universities with smoke-free air policies; 2011. Available at: http://no-smoke.org/pdf/smokefreecolleges universities.pdf. Accessed May 24, 2011.
35. Hopkins DP, Razi S, Leeks KD, et al. Smokefree policies to reduce tobacco use. A systematic review. Am J Prev Med 2010;38(Suppl 2):S275–89.
36. Lee JG, Goldstein AO, Kramer KD, et al. Statewide diffusion of 100% tobacco-free college and university policies. Tob Control 2010;19(4):311–7.
37. Berg CJ, Lessard L, Parelkar PP, et al. College student reactions to smoking bans in public, on campus and at home. Health Educ Res 2011;26(1):106–18.
38. Rigotti NA, Regan S, Moran SE, et al. Students' opinion of tobacco control policies recommended for US colleges: a national survey. Tob Control 2003;12(3):251–6.
39. Thompson B, Coronado GD, Chen L, et al. Preferred smoking policies at 30 Pacific Northwest colleges. Public Health Rep 2006;121(5):586–93.
40. American Lung Association. Big tobacco on campus: ending the addiction. Washington, DC: American Lung Association; 2008.
41. Rigotti NA, Moran SE, Wechsler H. US college students' exposure to tobacco promotions: prevalence and association with tobacco use. Am J Public Health 2005;95(1):138–44.
42. Stead LF, Bergson G, Lancaster T. Physician advice for smoking cessation. Cochrane Database Syst Rev 2008;2:CD000165.
43. Stead LF, Perera R, Bullen C, et al. Nicotine replacement therapy for smoking cessation. Cochrane Database Syst Rev 2008;1:CD000146.
44. Hughes JR, Stead LF, Lancaster T. Antidepressants for smoking cessation. Cochrane Database Syst Rev 2007;1:CD000031.
45. Ahluwalia JS, Okuyemi K, Nollen N, et al. The effects of nicotine gum and counseling among African American light smokers: a 2 × 2 factorial design. Addiction 2006;101(6):883–91.
46. American College Health Association. American College Health Association-National College Health Assessment II: reference group executive summary fall 2010. Linthicum (MD): American College Health Association; 2010.
47. Johnston L, O'Malley P, Bachman JG, et al. Monitoring the Future national survey results on drug use, 1975-2008. College students and adults ages 19–50. Bethesda (MD): National Institute on Drug Abuse; 2010.
48. National Institutes of Health. Panel says effective strategies to stop smoking are underused. Research Matters 2006. Available at. http://www.nih.gov/researchmatters/june2006/06232006smoking.htm. Accessed October 13, 2011.
49. Ridner SL, Hahn EJ. The pros and cons of cessation in college-age smokers. Clin Excell Nurse Pract 2005;9(2):81–7.

50. Velicer W, Prochaska J. A comparison of four self-report smoking cessation outcome measures. Addict Behav 2004;29(1):51–60.
51. Ockene J, Mermelstein R, Bonollo D, et al. Relapse and maintenance issues for smoking cessation. Health Psychol 2000;19(Suppl 1):17–31.
52. Agboola S, McNeill A, Coleman T, et al. A systematic review of the effectiveness of smoking relapse prevention interventions for abstinent smokers. Addiction 2010;105(8):1362–80.
53. Hajek P, Stead L, West R, et al. Relapse prevention interventions for smoking cessation. Cochrane Database Syst Rev 2009;1:CD003999.
54. Koontz J, Harris K, Okuyemi K, et al. Healthcare providers' treatment of college smokers. J Am Coll Health 2004;53(3):117–25.
55. Lawrance KA, Lawler SA. Campus physicians' tobacco interventions with university students: a descriptive study of 16 Ontario university clinics. Patient Educ Couns 2008;70(2):187–92.
56. Fagan K. Smoking-cessation counseling practices of college/university healthcare providers—a theory-based approach. J Am Coll Health 2007;55(6):351–9.
57. Wechsler H, Kelley K, Seibring M, et al. College smoking policies and smoking cessation programs: results of a survey of college health center directors. J Am Coll Health 2001;49(5):205–12.

# An Evidence-Based Cessation Strategy Using Rural Smokers' Experiences with Tobacco

Karen M. Butler, DNP, RN[a],*, Susan Hedgecock, MSN, RN[b],
Rachael A. Record, MA[b], Stephanie Derifield, MS[c],
Carolyn McGinn, MS, RD[d], Deborah Murray, EdD[e],
Ellen J. Hahn, PhD, RN[f]

**KEYWORDS**

- Rural adults • Tobacco cessation • Personal narratives
- Smoking cessation • Rural health

Tobacco use is the major cause of preventable disease and death in the United States, contributing to nearly 500,000 premature deaths annually.[1] More than 46 million US adults are current smokers (20.6%). Despite increasing efforts to provide tobacco-related programming and cessation assistance, the adult smoking prevalence did not change significantly from 2005 to 2009, suggesting a lull in the slight decline during the past decade.

Funding statement: the development of the HEEL program was made possible by Senator Mitch McConnell with funds earmarked for the University of Kentucky, College of Agriculture, Lexington, KY, and budgeted through the CSREES/USDA Federal Administration.
This publication was supported by grant number UL1RR033173 from the National Center for Research Resources (NCRR), funded by the Office of the Director, National Institutes of Health (NIH) and supported by the NIH Roadmap for Medical Research (E. Hahn and M.K. Rayens, Co-Investigators). The content is solely the responsibility of the authors and does not necessarily represent the official views of NCRR and NIH.
[a] College of Nursing, University of Kentucky, 423 CON Building, Lexington, KY 40536, USA
[b] College of Nursing, University of Kentucky, 509 CON Building, Lexington, KY 40536, USA
[c] Agriculture Extension, University of Kentucky, Lawrence County Extension Office, 249 Industrial Park Road, Louisa, KY 41230, USA
[d] Lawrence County Health Department, 1080 Meadowbrook Lane, Louisa, KY 41230, USA
[e] Health Education through Extension Leadership, School of Human Environmental Sciences/FCS, University of Kentucky, 1 Quality Street, Lexington, KY 40507, USA
[f] Tobacco Policy Research Program, Kentucky Center for Smoke-free Policy, University of Kentucky College of Nursing, 751 Rose Street, Lexington, KY 40536-0232, USA
* Corresponding author.
*E-mail address:* Karen.Butler@uky.edu

The burden of tobacco use in the United States is not evenly distributed. Nationally, higher smoking rates are found among men (23.5% vs 17.9% in women), as well as those with less than a high school diploma (28.5%) and those living below the federal poverty level (31.1%) or in the South (21.8%) and Midwest (23.1%).[1] According to the National Interview Survey (2007), national adult smoking prevalence among persons living in nonmetropolitan areas is 24.5%, higher than either the prevalence for small metro areas (20.9%) or large metro areas (17.4%).[2]

Rural smoking prevalence rates vary by state. Kentucky, a tobacco-growing state, is a national leader in rural adult smoking prevalence at 31.8%, which is higher than the state and national averages and the rates found in rural areas of other states. For example, rural areas of Utah have a much lower level of adult smoking prevalence, at 12.5%.[3] Low socioeconomic status (as measured by educational level, income, and employment) was associated with higher smoking prevalence in a national rural study and explained part of the disparity in tobacco use among rural residents. Regardless of location, rural populations are disproportionately affected by tobacco use, exposure to secondhand smoke, and smoking-attributable disease and death.[4]

Little is known about specific behavioral interventions that could enhance success rates among those who want to quit smoking, particularly those living in rural areas who are at higher risk and have less access to health care.[5] Nationally, most (70%) adult smokers report that they want to quit completely.[6] In 2008, an estimated 20.8 million (45.3%) adult smokers had tried to quit and had stopped smoking for at least 1 day during the preceding 12 months.[7] Although interventions designed to reach populations may have the greatest chance of success when they are tailored toward those at highest risk, they may not be as effective in rural areas because of limited access to health care.[5] However, innovative approaches have been tested in rural areas, including telephone counseling,[8] Web-based interventions,[9] and cessation contests.[10]

Unique cultural and social factors that exist in rural communities may affect tobacco use and treatment. For example, some communities may have social norms supportive of tobacco use (ie, tobacco-growing communities), or be exposed to tobacco industry marketing campaigns such as sponsorships of rural sporting events. Proximity to tobacco growing in rural areas is another potential barrier to tobacco control efforts.[5] Tobacco-growing regions of the country often have fewer tobacco-related laws and fewer antismoking programs.[11] However, all rural areas are not alike. Interventions that work well in one rural area may not necessarily translate to other rural areas.

Although rural communities are diverse, residents of rural communities tend to have strong family ties and close-knit social networks.[12,13] Participation in local organizations is high and neighborliness is valued. Tobacco interventions that tap into existing social networks, engage stakeholders, and gain the trust of rural residents could bridge the tobacco treatment gap in rural areas.[5] Because rural smokers are a population with a high potential for behavior change resistance, low levels of perceived vulnerability, and opposing social norms, they are an ideal population for an intervention based on the findings from personal narratives.[14]

Personal narratives are an innovative approach to reaching smokers in rural communities and motivating them to consider quitting. Hinyard and Kreuter[14] found that personal narratives are effective because they are personal, relatable, believable, and memorable. They cited 3 major reasons why personal narratives are effective: (1) the ability to reduce counterarguments, (2) the facilitation of observational learning, and (3) the ability to identify with the storyteller. Personal narratives have been used successfully with vulnerable populations to decrease tobacco, alcohol, and marijuana use[15–17] and show promise as an intervention to reach rural smokers to motivate them to think about quitting.[18] Personal narratives from members of vulnerable populations are successful at encouraging behavior change because other members of those populations can more easily relate to the given message[19] and have been shown to be an acceptable, culturally competent, and effective way to reach populations to promote healthy behaviors.[14,20]

The use of personal narratives to motivate rural smokers to think about quitting is supported by the literature, and is innovative and timely. Therefore, this article describes the personal narratives of current and former smokers living in an economically distressed, rural area of Appalachian Kentucky. It identifies themes and develops messages based on the collected personal narratives that could be used in designing messages and interventions to motivate smokers to make a quit attempt.[18] Data gathered in this research could potentially form the basis for culturally sensitive, cost-effective, population-based tobacco cessation interventions designed to reach rural smokers. The goal is to improve health outcomes through decreased tobacco use and exposure to secondhand smoke in this high-risk population. This outcome would in turn cut health care costs, reduce the number of illnesses requiring hospitalization as well as premature deaths, and improve the overall health of rural communities.

## METHODS

This was an exploratory focus group study using a qualitative approach to discover themes applicable to the design of future interventions. Qualitative interviews were used to elicit stories from current and recent former smokers. Current smokers were defined as those who had smoked at least 1 cigarette in the past 30 days; recent former smokers were those who had not smoked in the past 30 days.

Participants were invited to attend 1 of 3 scheduled focus group sessions held in different communities located in an economically distressed county in the Eastern Coalfield Region of Appalachian Kentucky (**Table 1**). Counties are designated as distressed based on 4 indicators: income, unemployment, poverty, and infant mortality. Distressed counties have a median family income no greater than two-thirds of the national average and a poverty rate that is at least 1.5 times the national average.[21] In addition, the county is medically underserved, characterized as having too few primary care providers, high infant mortality, high poverty, and/or large elderly population.[22]

Focus group participants were provided with a meal and childcare to encourage attendance. Attendees were also given a $15 gasoline card as an incentive to

**Table 1**
**Sociodemographic characteristics of the study county compared with state and national characteristics**

| Demographic | Study County | Kentucky | United States |
|---|---|---|---|
| Population[29] | 16,443 | 4,269,245 | 307,006,550 |
| White/African American (%)[29] | 98.7/0.3 | 89.9/7.7 | 79.8/12.8 |
| Median household income ($)[29] | 29,015 | 41,489 | 52,029 |
| Per capita income ($)[29] | 12,008 | 18,093 | 21,587 |
| Persons below poverty level (%)[29] | 27.1 | 17.3 | 13.2 |
| High school graduates (%)[29] | 58.2 | 74.1 | 80.4 |
| Adult smoking prevalence (%)[30] | 31.0 | 25.3 | 20.6 |

participate. Focus group sessions were facilitated by a graduate research assistant experienced in qualitative methods. An observer took field notes at all focus group sessions. All sessions were recorded using 2 tape recorders. Debriefing between the group leader and observer occurred immediately after each focus group.

### Sample

Current and former smokers (N = 21) were recruited via referrals from community key informants and by posting recruitment fliers throughout the county. There was a close collaboration with the county Cooperative Extension Agents and the health department tobacco control specialist in identifying both potential participants and recruitment flier locations. Participants were 100% white and 79% women. The mean age was 51.3 years (range 30–67 years); 81% had high school education or higher. Forty percent were employed outside the home; 25% were homemakers and 35% were disabled or retired. The mean age of smoking initiation was 14.4 years (range 6–21 years), and the mean number of years they had smoked was 31 (range 8–50 years). Thirty-seven percent had not smoked in the past 30 days before the focus group. Eighty-six percent had tried to quit smoking in the past. Sociodemographic characteristics of the study county, compared with state and national characteristics, are shown in **Table 1**.

### Interview Guide

The facilitator used a semistructured interview guide that included broad open-ended questions and a series of possible follow-up prompts (**Box 1** shows some sample questions). Questions were designed to capture respondents' personal narratives about tobacco use and to gain insights for the design of future tobacco interventions. Throughout the focus group sessions, the facilitator used motivational interviewing techniques, including reflection and restating, to verify statements made by participants and to encourage expansion of ideas.

---

**Box 1**
**Focus group interview guide sample questions**

1. Tell us about your county and community. What are some of the things that you like most about living where you do?

2. Please describe your first experience with tobacco.

   a. What were your feelings about tobacco then, and now?

   b. How might your past or present experiences with tobacco be different from those of people who do not live where you do?

3. Please tell us about a time a time when you tried to quit using tobacco.

   a. What people helped you the most in deciding to quit?

   b. What words did they use to help you?

4. Tell us things that you think would help people to make a decision to quit using tobacco in your county.

   a. Which of those things were most important to you to when you decided that you wanted to quit?

   b. If your best friend were using tobacco, how would you go about encouraging them to quit? What words would you use?

## Data Analysis

Recorded focus group sessions were transcribed for analysis, and the transcript was reviewed several times. Notes from the focus groups formed an early coding system that was checked with members of the research team for inter-rater reliability. Transcribed interviews were uploaded into Atlas.ti 6 software, and coded using the initial coding system as a reference. Codes were added as necessary to generate a complete coding system, which was again checked by the research team. Inter-rater reliability was 80%.

Using the code-quotation count feature in Atlas.ti 6, frequently occurring codes in the text were identified and reviewed for meaning. Codes of similar meanings were grouped, using the family manager feature. Families or themes from the grouped codes were interpreted and named. Themes and associated quotations were presented to the research team for feedback. In addition, the themes were presented to a small subset of the original focus group participants to verify accuracy.

## RESULTS

Nine focus group themes emerged from 357 data bits (**Table 2**). The top themes, in order of prevalence were: (1) need for easy access to tobacco dependence treatment, (2) quitting with support of family and friends, (3) faith, (4) quitting for health reasons, (5) freedom of individual choice, (6) pride of place, (7) Big Tobacco (ie, the tobacco industry, including the larger tobacco companies), (8) meaningful messages to smokers, and (9) quitting for one's children.

### Need for Easy Access to Tobacco Dependence Treatment

Participants voiced a willingness to try pharmaceutical aids in an effort to quit smoking, but stated that the cost was prohibitive. Prescription medications would be used if insurance covered the cost. In addition, cessation programs offering assistance with nicotine patches were cited as a motivation to quit.

One participant said, "Incentives like our boxes that we got. I can't go out and afford to buy a $35 box of patches. Or $30 or however much they are; that to me was a big lure" (to attend a tobacco dependence treatment program).

### Quitting with Support of Family and Friends

Participants stated that it was helpful to have the support of family and/or friends when making a quit attempt. Participants said: "I need my best friend to basically do it together at the same time (quit smoking), and I know it would be successful"; "If you want your best friend to quit, then you quit with them if you're a smoker," and "Even if it's just me and the 3 of us going 'How did you do today?'" (group of smokers supporting each other).

### Faith

Faith was both a motivator and a positive force when they were trying to quit smoking. A desire to please God motivated 1 respondent to quit smoking. "I was on my way to church one morning and I wanted a closer relationship with God and it was almost as though He physically said, until you leave those alone, we can't go any farther...I haven't smoked since...I really think that for Christ we will do things that we wouldn't do for anybody else." Another stated: "... I really believe if you quit for some other reason, you're going to fail at it because there's one thing stronger than anything else and that's the God of wonder."

**Table 2**
**Focus group themes, sample quotes, and data bits**

| Focus Group Themes | Number of Data Bits | Percent of Total |
|---|---|---|
| Need for easy access to tobacco dependence treatment programs "The Health Department having that program where the patches were so cheap…that's wonderful to me…that they cared enough about their citizens." | 61 | 17 |
| Quitting with support of family and friends "My husband and I tried to quit smoking one time at the same time. …he said, I don't think I can do this. I said, yeah we can." | 59 | 17 |
| Faith "I know that when the good Lord up above feels that I'm ready to do it, He'll help me through it." | 55 | 15 |
| Quitting for health reasons "As I get older and my breathing is affected and I just had bronchitis for the third time…know something's gotta change." | 42 | 12 |
| Freedom of individual choice "I don't think that the government should come along and tell me or my friend that lives over the hill over here that's a tobacco farmer…that I can't smoke in the city…something sticks in my craw about that." | 36 | 10 |
| Pride of place "We have more talent in this area, in this river, up and down this river…the most beautiful quilts you've ever saw, some woodworking, you know, I mean there's talent here." | 33 | 9 |
| Big Tobacco "I don't know what they're putting in them things that are so addictive and I think it's more addictive in the last 15 to 20 years than it ever was." | 27 | 8 |
| Meaningful messages to smokers "Telling me to quit, you just need to quit, that's not support to me…being able to understand what I'm going through." | 26 | 7 |
| Quitting for one's children "My grandson said, oh Mamaw, you stopped smoking so I won't get so sick anymore. And I thought, oh my God, you know. You don't realize how they see it and it was like, oh praise the Lord, I never go back." | 18 | 5 |
| Total | 357 | 100 |

## Quitting for Health Reasons

Participants cited acute and chronic health problems as reasons to quit. Several voiced relief with improved health after quitting smoking: "I don't even feel like I smoked before. I feel cleaner. I treated myself to new perfume just because I felt so much better. I breathe better; I don't take my asthma and my allergy medicine. I just feel 100% better and that's like a treat to me, I treated myself to that," and "I don't cough when I laugh anymore. I used to; every time I'd start to laugh, man, a big old cough would come out."

Conversely, some said that experience with other people's illness caused them to smoke more: "Watching her try to breathe... I thought about stopping but then it turns out that I ended up smoking more after she died, which I couldn't understand... I'm watching this poor lady die because she can't breathe and instead of quitting, I just smoked more."

### Freedom of Individual Choice

Both current and recent former smokers stated that others should not intrude on their right to choose to smoke or not smoke and that smoking should be an individual choice: "...I really don't think it's any of my business if they smoke; I choose not to." Another stated: "I agree...that it's a choice... I made my choice." Some respondents voiced resentment at smoking restrictions: "No, I don't have the greatest habit in the world...but nor am I illiterate or a criminal because I smoke." Others made statements related to readiness to quit smoking that strongly supported freedom of individual choice: "When you're ready, when it hurts bad enough you'll change it," and "For me, it got to be a burden, the cigarette you know. I had to be ready. I'm just thankful I don't have to worry about that burden anymore."

### Pride of Place

Participants voiced great pride in their community, and stated that they resent negative stereotypes about Appalachia. Many spoke of the natural beauty of their surroundings, the talents of the people, and the feelings of closeness with family, friends, and people within community organizations. "...It's very pretty. And I enjoy my church, which is right here, and the people...I really do enjoy where I live," and "What I like about it I think is the closeness...of the communities and friends. It's a lovely place to live."

### Big Tobacco

Participants' views of the tobacco industry were ambivalent. There were sympathetic views toward tobacco farmers, and feelings that the tobacco fields were beautiful.

"I think the tobacco fields are beautiful...when it's topping out and just getting ready to be cut down, it's just so pretty." One said "To look at tobacco in the fields... to me it doesn't say cigarettes."

Some voiced suspicions of the cigarette manufacturers, who they thought were deliberately trying to addict and hold on to smokers as customers: "I really think that these companies are...trying to keep us their customers. They don't want us to go away and they'll do anything they can do."

Others voiced similar beliefs related to the addictiveness of nicotine: "I don't know what's in it but now it's a little devil that pulls you back and it is so hard, it gets a hold of you and there it is" (on what's in cigarettes and trying to quit), and "I'm not addicted to drugs but I'm addicted to nicotine."

### Meaningful Messages to Smokers

Current and recent former smokers stated that helpful messages to smokers during a cessation attempt should come from former smokers, and that others should be supportive of the smoker's decision to smoke or not smoke. One stated "...the only real support system that anybody could have as a smoker or even an addict is somebody that's been there themselves. If you've not smoked, you're not going to be a supporter for me because you don't know what I'm going through." Another suggested message was "Do it because you want to, not because someone says you have to....that's good. Be supportive and not judgmental." Others suggested that helpful messages may be "Let's do it together" (quitting smoking), and "I never felt myself breathe that well since I was a teenager" (what you would tell your best friend trying to quit).

### Quitting for One's Children

Children or grandchildren and the desire to either set an example for them or not expose them to secondhand smoke were frequently mentioned as motivation to quit.

One parent said, "Well my children…and being pregnant was my first 2 influences to try to quit smoking…my youngest daughter…was a thumb sucker and she said, 'Mommy I will quit sucking my thumb if you'll quit smoking; fair trade.' So I quit…the only [thing]…that matters to me is my children."

Others voiced similar concerns: "I have 1 granddaughter that's allergic to it [smoke] and if she's around it very much then she has to get on the breathing machine," and "My son, you know, he said, 'Mommy are you smoking again?' I know that I shouldn't smoke around him but I do. I want to quit. I know I can but you know there is just something there that draws you and it's addiction."

## DISCUSSION

The 9 focus group themes can be classified into 3 groups: (1) personal motivators to quit smoking, (2) external influences, and (3) pride of place. Most of these themes are consistent with the findings of similar research conducted in Appalachia[23–29] and with rural or disparate populations,[3,10,30,31] but there are novel ideas that offer intriguing insights and implications for further research and intervention development in rural communities.

### Personal Motivators to Quit Smoking

Rural smokers and recent former smokers said that health concerns and their children affected their smoking and decisions to quit. Our findings indicate that chronic illnesses can be both a motivator to quit smoking as well as a stressor that could deter cessation. This dichotomy is similar to the findings of Hutcheson and colleagues,[31] who found that illness could both prompt thoughts about quitting and generate stress that led to continued smoking among a sample of rural Kansans. Similarly, Rayens and colleagues[10] found that a major illness could influence readiness to quit smoking. However, in a study of smoking relatives of patients with lung cancer, 91% of smoking family members still smoked following an educational intervention about the benefits of smoking cessation.[32]

Our finding that concern for children as a motivator to quit to smoking is supported by other studies of rural populations. Appalachian respondents reported a desire to protect children from tobacco use in focus groups held in 7 states.[27] A desire to set a good example for children and protect them from secondhand smoke was a facilitator of smoking cessation in rural Kansans.[31] Burgess and colleagues[30] found that, in a study of rural American Indians, women felt guilt and pressure to quit when smoking around children. This guilt was also echoed in statements from focus group participants in the study reported here.

Study results also revealed a strong theme of independence and a desire to be allowed the freedom to make choices. This finding is consistent with research that shows personal independence, individualism, self-reliance, and price to be important in Appalachian culture. Our findings are similar to those of Ahijevych and colleagues,[23] who examined beliefs about tobacco use and cessation among current and former tobacco users in rural Appalachia. Our participants spoke of resenting smoke-free restrictions, which they thought impinged on their rights to choose, stating that they were offended at being treated like a criminal. Hutcheson and colleagues[31] found that smoking restrictions engendered similar sentiments of feeling like a second-class citizen, but were also a facilitator of smoking cessation. Hahn and colleagues[33] reported that adult smoking prevalence decreased after enactment of a comprehensive smoke-free law. In our study, it is unclear whether negative feelings about smoking restrictions were related to quit attempts, although some expressed the positive benefits of cessation related to smoking restrictions. Although smoking restrictions could also be considered external influences, the strongest part of this theme was consistent with the personal desire to make choices for oneself.

Our study offers some new insights regarding the role of faith in quitting smoking. Although the tie between religious faith and health in Appalachia,[24–26,28] and between faith and addiction,[34] has been documented, our study adds a more detailed description of how faith might motivate some smokers to quit. Specifically, we found that the desire to please God with one's life and the belief that God would help the smoker through the quitting process were expressed by participants as motivational. Integrating tobacco dependence treatment into the faith community may be an effective reach strategy in rural communities.

## External Influences on Smoking

Participants expressed the importance of ease of access to tobacco dependence treatment, quitting with the support of family and friends, and the influence of Big Tobacco, and they suggested messages that might be most effective in helping smokers quit. Easy access to treatment is difficult in rural areas, which typically lack public transportation and access to childcare, as well as other social and health services. Unemployment rates, poverty levels, low rates of health insurance, and poor availability of health care are barriers to rural smokers who wish to seek tobacco dependence treatment.[3,31] Although rural Kansans were willing to try pharmacologic approaches to cessation, cost was a barrier.[31] Similarly, our study revealed that easy access to tobacco dependence treatment was appreciated by the participants, and that they took advantage of cessation services that were either free or provided at reduced cost.

Our study identified quitting with the support of family and friends to be a dominant theme, which is consistent with other studies.[35] Appalachian culture is family centered, with a social structure that is based on kinship. Social support from family and friends was an important factor in making health-related decisions.[23,25] Rayens and colleagues[10] found that positive partner support increased readiness to quit smoking among rural Kentuckians. Song and Fish[29] found an association between partner support and nonsmoking among pregnant women in Appalachian West Virginia.

Although there was much pride voiced in this rural community and its people, no connection was drawn between tobacco use and tobacco growing. Meyer and colleagues[27] also reported such a cognitive disconnect between growing tobacco and the harm of tobacco use in the minds of farmers, with respondents stating that farmers are not thinking about tobacco smoking when they are growing it. Ambivalence about tobacco was evident. Although none of the participants in our study grew tobacco, they expressed sympathetic views toward tobacco farming. Suspicion and negative views were voiced toward the cigarette manufacturers, or Big Tobacco. The beauty of the growing tobacco fields was not associated with the production or smoking of cigarettes in their responses.

Regarding messages that might be meaningful to smokers, it was important for our participants to know that the person giving the message was a current or former smoker, and that the message be nonjudgmental. The notion that other current or former smokers may be more effective at supporting quit attempts is not found commonly in the literature, and can be used when designing culturally appropriate interventions for this population. The notion that messages should be nonjudgmental is well supported in the literature. For example, Falomir-Pichastor and colleagues[36] found it essential for messages to be respectful toward smokers. Disrespectful messages can cause one to get defensive and, in return, become less receptive. Creating messages based on information gathered through personal narratives can help ensure the creation of respectful messages and therefore increase the receptiveness of the audience.

Our participants also identified relationships with, and messages from, family and friends as an important factor when trying to quit smoking. This finding is supported by Ahijevych and colleagues,[23] who found evidence of the importance of family and personal independence in relation to tobacco use. Meyer and colleagues[27] found that tobacco education in Appalachia acknowledges the central role of the family, and that messages tailored to cultural themes may decrease prevalence.

The meaningful messages theme also revealed an interconnectedness with other themes that provides direction in devising the main messages that may be effective with rural smokers. The messages identified as most meaningful to those wanting to quit smoking included statements that support the importance of individual choice (quitting when you are ready, not because someone else says you should), support from family and friends (quitting together), and quitting for health reasons. This overlap between themes has implications for appropriately framing a culturally sensitive message that may be meaningful in motivating rural smokers to consider quitting.

### Pride of Place

Pride of place was a strong theme heard throughout all 3 focus groups. There was great admiration and pride voiced for the famous people who were born and raised in the area (ie, country music singers, elected officials, movie stars) and in the talents and products of the local crafts artists (ie, quilting, woodworking). Prior research has confirmed this finding of loyalty to place among Appalachian residents.[13] There is a collective identity that is bound up in community and place of worship and creates great pride in both neighbors and community. This finding may be important in the use of personal narratives as vehicles for tobacco control messages. Messages that are respectful of community traditions may have greater reception than those that do not contain this element.[13]

### SUMMARY

This article describes the personal narratives of current and recent former smokers living in an economically distressed rural area of Kentucky. Rural smokers face unique challenges in that there is often lack of resources, resulting in barriers to accessing evidence-based tobacco dependence treatment. It is important that tobacco control resources and efforts be allocated appropriately so that smokers living in rural, economically distressed communities have easy access to evidence-based tobacco dependence treatment. Because 20% to 25% of the US population lives in rural communities and their smoking rates are disproportionately high, it is important to address the unique needs of rural smokers.[31] Identifying the personal narratives and messages of rural smokers is important when considering how best to tailor both reach and efficacy interventions to meet their needs related to smoking cessation.

A potential limitation of the study is that the sample was small and participant selection was not random. These findings are not intended to be generalizable to other populations. An additional potential limitation is that this study was funded by earmark money, which may be interpreted by some as a conflict of interest. This study was conducted in accordance with scientific principles without influence from others, including the funders of the study.

Further research is needed to examine fidelity, acceptability, practicality, and reach of culturally sensitive interventions developed from the personal narratives and messages. The effects of these culturally sensitive reach interventions need to be tested on enrollment and attendance in tobacco dependence treatment, and on nicotine dependence and cessation outcomes.

Capturing messages from personal narratives represents an evidence-based, data-rich strategy for the development of culturally sensitive, population-based interventions for rural smokers. Use of personalized, culturally sensitive strategies may be effective in reaching rural smokers and motivating them to quit, thereby reducing tobacco-related disease and death in economically distressed rural communities.

## REFERENCES

1. Dube S, McClave A, Caraballo R, et al. Vital signs: current cigarette smoking among adults aged = 18 years—United States, 2009. MMWR Morb Mortal Wkly Rep 2010;59:1135–40.
2. Pleis JR, Lucas JW. Summary health statistics for US adults: National Health Interview Survey, 2007. Vital Health Stat 10 2009;(240):1.
3. Doescher MP, Jackson JE, Jerant AL, et al. Prevalence and trends in smoking: a national rural study. J Rural Health 2006;22(2):112–8.
4. Rahilly C, Farwell W. Prevalence of smoking in the United States: a focus on age, sex, ethnicity, and geographic patterns. Curr Cardiovasc Risk Rep 2007;1(5): 379–83.
5. Tobacco control in rural America. Washington DC: American Legacy Foundation; 2009.
6. Centers for Disease Control and Prevention. Cigarette smoking among adult—United States, 2001. MMWR Morb Mortal Wkly Rep 2003;52(40):953–5.
7. Centers for Disease Control and Prevention. Cigarette smoking among adults and trends in smoking cessation–United States, 2008. MMWR Morb Mortal Wkly Rep 2009;58(44):1227–32.
8. Cox LS, Cupertino AP, Mussulman LM, et al. Design and baseline characteristics from the KAN-QUIT disease management intervention for rural smokers in primary care. Prev Med 2008;47(2):200–5.
9. Stoops WW, Dallery J, Fields NM, et al. An Internet-based abstinence reinforcement smoking cessation intervention in rural smokers. Drug Alcohol Depend 2009;105(1–2):56–62.
10. Rayens MK, Hahn E, Hedgecock S. Readiness to quit smoking in rural communities. Issues Ment Health Nurs 2008;29:1115–33.
11. Hahn EJ, Toumey CP, Rayens MK, et al. Kentucky legislators' views on tobacco policy. Am J Prev Med 1999;16(2):81–8.
12. Bauer WM, Growick B. Rehabilitation counseling in Appalachian America. J Rehabil 2003;69(3):18–24.

13. Schoenberg NE, Hatcher J, Dignan MB. Appalachian women's perceptions of their community's health threats. J Rural Health 2008;24(1):75–83.

14. Hinyard LJ, Kreuter MW. Using narrative communication as a tool for health behavior change: a conceptual, theoretical, and empirical overview. Health Educ Behav 2007;34(5):777.

15. Horn K, McCracken L, Dino G, et al. Applying community-based participatory research principles to the development of a smoking-cessation program for American Indian teens: "Telling our story". Health Educ Behav 2008;35:44–69.

16. Horn K, McGloin T, Dino G, et al. Quit and reduction rates for a pilot study of the American Indian Not On Tobacco (NOT) program. Prev Chronic Dis 2005; 2(4):A13.

17. Nelson A, Arthur B. Storytelling for empowerment: decreasing at-risk youth's alcohol and marijuana use. J Prim Prev 2003;24:169–80.

18. Rollins E, Terrion JL. Explorations of self-efficacy: personal narratives as qualitative data in the analysis of smoking cessation efforts. J Smok Cessat 2010;5(1): 57–68.

19. Dal Cin S, Zanna MP, Fong GT, Linn JA. Narrative persuasion and overcoming resistance. In: Knowles ES, editor. Resistance and persuasion. Mahwah (NJ): Lawrence Erlbaum and Associates; 2004. p. 175–91.

20. Hodge F, Pasqua A, Marquez C, et al. Utilizing traditional storytelling to promote wellness in American Indian communities. J Transcult Nurs 2002;13:6–11.

21. County economic status and distressed areas in the Appalachian region, fiscal year 2009. Washington, DC: Appalachian Regional Commission; 2008.

22. Shortage designation: health professional shortage areas & medically underserved areas/populations. US Department of Health and Human Services; 2011.

23. Ahijevych K, Kuun P, Christman S, et al. Beliefs about tobacco among Appalachian current and former users. Appl Nurs Res 2003;16(2):93–102.

24. Barish R, Snyder AE. Use of complementary and alternative healthcare practices among persons served by a remote area medical clinic. Fam Community Health 2008;31(3):221.

25. Coyne CA, Demian-Popescu C, Friend D. Social and cultural factors influencing health in southern West Virginia: a qualitative study. Prev Chronic Dis 2006;3(4): A124.

26. Jesse DE, Reed PG. Effects of spirituality and psychosocial well being on health risk behaviors in Appalachian pregnant women. J Obstet Gynecol Neonatal Nurs 2004;33(6):739–47.

27. Meyer MG, Toborg MA, Denham SA, et al. Cultural perspectives concerning adolescent use of tobacco and alcohol in the Appalachian mountain region. J Rural Health 2008;24(1):67–74.

28. Simpson MR, King MG. "God brought all these churches together": issues in developing religion health partnerships in an Appalachian community. Public Health Nurs 1999;16(1):41–9.

29. Song H, Fish M. Demographic and psychosocial characteristics of smokers and nonsmokers in low socioeconomic status rural Appalachian 2-parent families in southern West Virginia. J Rural Health 2006;22(1):83–7.

30. Burgess D, Fu SS, Joseph AM, et al. Beliefs and experiences regarding smoking cessation among American Indians. Nicotine Tob Res 2007;9:19–28.

31. Hutcheson TD, Greiner KA, Ellerbeck EF, et al. Understanding smoking cessation in rural communities. J Rural Health 2008;24(2):116–24.

32. Schilling A, Conaway MR, Wingate PJ, et al. Recruiting cancer patients to participate in motivating their relatives to quit smoking. Cancer 1997;79(1):152–60.

33. Hahn EJ, Rayens MK, Butler KM, et al. Smoke-free laws and adult smoking prevalence. Prev Med 2008;47(2):206–9.
34. Borras L, Khazaal Y, Khan R, et al. The relationship between addiction and religion and its possible implication for care. Subst Use Misuse 2010;45(14): 2357.
35. Fiore M, Jaén C, Baker T, et al. Treating tobacco use and dependence: 2008 update. Rockville (MD): US Department of Health and Human Services, Public Health Service; 2008.
36. Falomir-Pichastor JM, Invernizzi F, Mugny G, et al. Social influence on intention to quit smoking: the effect of the rhetoric of an identity relevant message. Revue Internationale de Psychologie Sociale 2002;15(1):81–96.

# Evidence-Based Tobacco Cessation Strategies with Pregnant Latina Women

Elizabeth Moran Fitzgerald, EdD, APRN, PMHCNS-BC

**KEYWORDS**

- Tobacco cessation • Pregnant • Hispanic/Latina • Women
- Evidence based

The prevalence of tobacco use in women is about 18% in the United States,[1] and most female smokers currently reside in developed countries.[2] The tobacco industry focuses its global marketing strategies on youth, lower socioeconomic populations, minorities, and developing countries.[3] According to the National Center for Health Statistics,[4] Hispanic pregnant women have lower rates of tobacco use (2.6%) as compared with blacks (8.4%) and whites (13.8%). However, the literature also suggests that rates of tobacco cessation by Hispanics during pregnancy are lower and their relapse rates during the postpartum period are higher.[5,6]

Smoking is an important cause of poor pregnancy outcomes in the United States and contributes to adverse outcomes, such as miscarriage, placental abruption and separation, premature rupture of membranes, preterm delivery, low birth weight, increased prenatal mortality, still birth, and sudden infant death syndrome.[7] According to the Centers for Disease Control and Prevention (CDC),[8] minority women are aware of the health risks associated with tobacco use and are motivated to quit. However, minority women also face significant hurdles to participate in tobacco cessation programs or to gain access to tobacco cessation resources.[9,10] Barriers to accessing care include a shortage of accessible health care providers, lack of insurance, lack of transportation and child care, immigration issues, language barriers, and other socio-cultural barriers.[11,12] Meta-analyses in the clinical literature have shown that mental health treatments, such as tobacco cessation counseling, are 4 times more effective when they are culturally modified for the specific target group and considerate of the cultural context and values.[13]

The 2010 census estimated that there were 50.5 million Hispanics in the United States, composing 16.3% of the total population. The Census Bureau also estimates

Lansing School of Nursing & Health Sciences, Bellarmine University, 2001 Newburg Road, Louisville, KY 40205, USA
E-mail address: efitzgerald@bellarmine.edu

Nurs Clin N Am 47 (2012) 45–54
doi:10.1016/j.cnur.2011.11.001                                  nursing.theclinics.com

there are 30.1 million Hispanic adults currently living in the United States, with 48% being women. According to the Pew Hispanic Center,[14,15] the number of Hispanics living in the United States grew 46.3% in the past decade, and overall growth in the Hispanic population accounted for most of the nation's growth from 2000 to 2010.

This review of the literature summarizes evidence-based practices for tobacco cessation among Latina women, with a focus on pregnant women and evidence-based practices that may hold promise for this population. Nurses who wish to use evidence-based practice interventions with pregnant Latina women must always be mindful of social and economic factors, social support networks, the physical and social environment, access to health services, and social and health policies when developing and planning tobacco cessation interventions in the community.

## THE HEALTHY MIGRANT EFFECT AND THE LATINA PARADOX

According to the Pew Hispanic Center,[16] Latinos are in relatively good health compared with other Americans. However, many Hispanics lack health insurance and regular health care. The Pew Hispanic Center report,[17] based on 2008 census data, stated Latinos are twice as likely as the overall US population to lack health insurance coverage, with approximately 50% of foreign-born Hispanics uninsured. According to Dubard and Gizlice,[18] Spanish-speaking US Hispanics were also more likely to have been unable to see a doctor for needed care because of cost. Spanish-speaking US Hispanics reported lower rates of tobacco use, physical activity, and binge drinking than English-speaking US Hispanics, as well as lower prevalence rates of arthritis, asthma, high blood pressure, and obesity. In this study, variances were not explained by differences in age, gender, and level of education. Dubard and Gizlice suggested a "healthy migrant" effect to explain this phenomenon.[18] The literature suggests that the US Spanish-speaking population is composed of immigrants who have recently migrated to the United States and are recognized as being in particularly good health. However, as Latino immigrants adopt the lifestyle of mainstream Americans and acculturate, they begin to acquire habits that lower their health status.[16] However, more research is needed to refine measures of acculturation,[19] including smoking, which is part of the social-cultural context and is influenced by sociocultural norms.[20] The literature suggests a negative influence of acculturation on tobacco use by Hispanic immigrants.[21]

Fleuriet[22] identified problems when using the concept of the Latina paradox with pregnant Latina women. In the literature, the Latina paradox attributes higher levels of social support with better-than-expected birth outcomes for babies of women who have emigrated from Mexico to the United States.[23] However, Fleuriet's analysis of qualitative data with 28 low-income immigrant women who migrated from Mexico to Texas determined that preferences for types of social support varied based on how a woman made meaning of her pregnancy. Fleuriet noted that epidemiologic research on the Latina paradox may be limited because of a presumption of cultural homogeneity among immigrant women of Mexican descent, an absence of cultural sensitivity in instruments used to measure social support during pregnancy, and a presumption that perception and availability of support indicate a woman's desire or intent to engage that support. The literature suggests that individualized treatment is needed to provide the optimal type, timing, and amount of social support for a particular person.[24]

## TOBACCO CESSATION INTERVENTIONS

Pregnancy presents a unique window of opportunity for positive health behavior change. According to the CDC,[8] women are more likely to quit smoking during pregnancy than at any other time in their life, and the clinical literature indicates that most pregnant women quit on discovery that they are pregnant. The term *spontaneous quitters* has been used to describe this phenomenon.[25]

Morasco, Dornelas, Fishcher, Oncken, and Lando[26] conducted a study of 141 low-income pregnant women who were predominately Hispanic and who stopped smoking without professional interventions. In this study, 33 Hispanic women (23% of the sample) were able to spontaneously quit smoking and they were then randomly assigned into 1 of 2 groups[1]: a psychotherapy relapse prevention treatment that included one 90-minute session followed by bimonthly phone calls during the pregnancy and monthly calls after delivery or[2] to usual care that provided an educational booklet on the importance of smoking cessation for pregnant women entitled, "Quitting for You 2." The addition of the psychotherapy relapse prevention intervention did not provide additional protection against relapse for the spontaneous quitters. The researchers concluded that most women who spontaneously quit smoking while pregnant will abstain from smoking at least until delivery.

The researchers recommended helpful interventions for spontaneous quitters, such as brief relapse-prevention counseling with a specific focus on the prevention of postpartum relapse to be delivered in the final trimester of pregnancy or after delivery. Their findings suggest the need for tobacco cessation programs to have a greater focus on the postpartum period when many women are more likely to resume smoking. Perhaps future studies could offer Hispanic pregnant women the relapse-prevention treatment in Spanish or English delivered by culturally sensitive providers to determine if this makes a difference.

### Nicotine Replacement Therapy

Women who are not able to spontaneously stop smoking during pregnancy, especially heavy smokers, may find it more difficult to quit. However, the safety of nicotine replacement therapies (NRT) during pregnancy needs additional research. Many health care providers are reluctant to prescribe NRT because of unknown pregnancy concerns. Gaither, Huber, Thompson, and Hudson[27] conducted a study to determine demographic characteristics of women who were prescribed or recommended NRT during pregnancy. They also investigated if the prescription or recommendation was related to adverse pregnancy outcomes. Their findings revealed that pregnant smokers less than 35 years of age and of Hispanic, non-Hispanic black, and Asian/Pacific Islander race or ethnicity were less likely to be prescribed or recommended NRT. The investigators also concluded that risks of low birth weight and preterm birth were highest for women who were prescribed or recommended NRT.

### Lay Health Advisors

The use of lay health advisor (LHA) programs has demonstrated beneficial outcomes with a variety of ethnic populations, including Hispanics.[28–30] Brief tobacco cessation interventions using lay persons as interventionists may impact a larger number of persons. The Institute of Medicine issued a call for the expansion of LHA programs to reduce health disparities in minority communities in 2002.[31] The use of lay advisors to provide tobacco cessation to Hispanic persons fits well with other community-based health intervention programs.

Campbell, Mays, Yuan, and Muramoto[30] conducted a study to describe the characteristics of lay health advisors in Arizona. The researchers recruited 910 lay health advisors and randomly assigned them to different training modalities. The analysis of the data revealed that advisors who have an interest in tobacco cessation may exhibit a combination of high motivation yet little knowledge of evidence-based tobacco cessation practices. Their findings showed that increasing the advisors' level of confidence was not as important as teaching them core knowledge concepts about tobacco interventions. The researchers think the use of LHAs has promise for tobacco cessation interventions in underserved minority communities and recommended more research to determine specific health influence behaviors.

Martinez-Bristow, Sias, Urquidi, and Feng[32] designed a model of tobacco cessation services using community health workers for Spanish-speaking populations in El Paso, Texas. They collaborated with the University of Arizona's HealthCare Partnership to train Spanish-speaking community health workers as tobacco cessation counselors. Tobacco Free El Paso certified the lay health workers to identify tobacco users and offer cessation-counseling services. Community health workers could choose to be certified at 3 levels: introductory, intermediate, and advanced. The results indicated that the community health workers acquired the appropriate level of knowledge and confidence to successfully offer tobacco cessation interventions in the community. Specific information about tobacco cessation during pregnancy could be added to the certification training courses to better prepare lay health workers to work with pregnant women.

Borrelli, McQuaid, Novak, Hammond, and Becker[33] studied Latino caregivers of children with asthma and conducted a randomized trial to motivate caregivers to quit smoking. Participants did not have to indicate a motivation to quit smoking to be in the study, they only had to be willing to agree to talk about their smoking and receive asthma education. Subjects were randomly assigned to receive 1 of 2 smoking-cessation interventions during a home-based asthma program[1]: a behavioral action model (BAM) based on clinical guidelines for tobacco cessation or[2] a precaution adoption model (PAM) based on feedback on the caregiver's carbon monoxide level and the child's secondhand smoke exposure using motivational interviewing. Only the PAM treatment was designed to be consistent with core Latino values, such as *personalismo*, *familismo*, and *simpatia*, yet both BAM and PAM interventions were delivered by a bilingual Latina health educator and counseling was provided in either English or Spanish.

The findings revealed that 20.5% of participants in the PAM condition and 9.1% of participants in the BAM condition were continuously abstinent at 2 months posttreatment. Findings also showed that 19.1% of participants in the PAM condition and 12.3% of those in the BAM condition were continuously abstinent at 3 months posttreatment. Children's asthma morbidity also declined significantly in the posttreatment period in the PAM group ($P<.05$). The findings support that incorporating Latino values into cessation programs is crucial to increase the likelihood of engaging Latinos in treatment.[34] Although this intervention program was not targeted specifically to Latino pregnant women, the study could be replicated with this population.

English and colleagues[11] designed, developed, and implemented an evidence-based perinatal tobacco cessation program for low-income women using LHAs. The intervention was delivered in a community-based, maternal and infant health program, and participants were predominately African American and Hispanic. The Hispanic population in this study consisted primarily of first-generation immigrants from El Salvador, Honduras, Costa Rica, and Mexico. The study's intervention was modeled on the evidence-based 5A's model endorsed by the US Public Health Service and the American College of Obstetricians and Gynecologists.[35] This best-practice model incorporates 5 simple steps and can be delivered in a relatively short time during patient-provider encounters. The researchers used the 5A's model as a starting point and then developed a brief scale to allow more-detailed response choices to tobacco use other than yes or no. Following the pilot testing period, the tobacco assessment forms were integrated into a more-structured protocol based on the 5A's model. A tool kit was given to the lay case managers to help them determine the client's smoking status, readiness for change, and the most appropriate tobacco cessation intervention.

English and colleagues[11] found 11% of the women who reported tobacco use during the intake quit smoking during their enrollment in the program. Although this quit rate was low, the researchers determined that the 5A's model was easy for LHAs to learn and that having a sustained commitment to training LHAs was important. These findings supported the literature that using a context-based approach is better to reduce racial, ethnic, and socioeconomic health disparities.

### Transtheoretical Model of Health Behavior Change

The transtheoretical model of health behavior change[36] has been used to support pregnant women who are trying to quit smoking. This model is safer than pharmacologic methods for smoking cessation by pregnant women and therefore health care providers may be more willing to recommend it for women who are not able to quit smoking spontaneously. Five dynamic stages compose the model and include pre-contemplation, contemplation, preparation, action, and maintenance.[37] Behavioral techniques are used by interventionists to guide the client through change. This model has been used in tobacco cessation programs with women and could easily be incorporated into programs for pregnant women who desire to stop smoking in a variety of settings. The model is can be taught to health care professionals and paraprofessionals.

### Timing of intervention during pregnancy

Yunzal-Butler, Joyce, and Racine[38] studied the association between the timing of enrollment in Women, Infants, and Children (WIC) and smoking among prenatal WIC participants. Their large sample size allowed the researchers to analyze smoking for non-Hispanic whites, non-Hispanic blacks, and Hispanics. The researchers found that participants who enrolled in WIC in the first or second trimester of pregnancy were more likely to quit than those who enrolled in the third trimester. The researchers recommended that WIC's role in smoking cessation should be strengthened to provide more focused counseling. One limitation to these findings is that Hispanic women and children who are undocumented may not be eligible for WIC services.

### Technology-Based and Telephonic Interventions

Social support for health behavior change, such as tobacco cessation, is frequently being provided by electronic technologies, including the Internet, text messaging, E-mail, and social networking.[39] However, according to the Pew Hispanic Center,[40] Latinos are less likely than Caucasians to access the Internet, own a home broadband connection, or own a cell phone. However, when socializing and communicating with friends, young Latinos (eg, aged 16–25 years) use mobile technology frequently. Fifty percent of young Latinos text message friends daily, so text messaging may be a useful strategy for the prevention of tobacco use or tobacco cessation with young

Latinos.[41] The use of text messaging for tobacco prevention and cessation should be replicated with pregnant Latina women.

Munoz, Barrerera, Delucchi, Penilla, Torres, and Perez-Stable[42] published the results of a randomized controlled trial that involved 500 Spanish-speaking and 500 English-speaking adult Internet users who were at least 18 years old, smoked at least 5 cigarettes daily, intended to quit in the next month, and used E-mail at least once a week. The participants were randomized into 4 interventions[1]: a National Cancer Institute evidence-based stop smoking guide[2]; intervention 1 plus E-mail reminders to return to the site,[3] condition 2 plus mood-management education; and[4] condition 3 plus a virtual group via an asynchronous bulletin board. Participants who consented to be in the study kept a log of the number of cigarettes smoked on 3 days within 1 week and set a quit date.

Outcomes were based on a self-report of 7-day abstinence rates at 1, 3, 6, and 12 months after the participant's initial quit date. The findings revealed no significant differences among the 4 conditions. The Spanish speakers' overall 12-month 7-day abstinence rates were 20.2% and English speakers were 21.0%. Although the English speakers' quit rates at 1, 3, and 6 months were slightly higher than the Spanish speakers' rates, the Spanish speakers' quit rates caught up to the English speakers' rates at the 12-month follow-up. These findings emphasize the importance of doing a follow-up beyond 6 months with Spanish-speaking populations. The researchers concluded that the Internet can allow health care providers to reach a wider audience of smokers than traditional tobacco cessation programs that provide face-to-face or pharmacologic interventions. They also recommended that their Internet tobacco cessation site (http://www.stopsmoking.ucsf.edu and http://www.dejardefumar.ucsf.edu) should be made available at no charge to users in a variety of languages and that national and international health organizations should help publicize tobacco cessation sites. Although the study did not indicate if any of the female participants were pregnant, future research with pregnant Latina women using Internet-based tobacco cessation programs may be warranted.

Burns and Levinson[43] studied the effects of a Spanish-language media campaign on the outcomes of a state-sponsored telephone quit line among Latino and non-Latino smokers in Colorado. Focus groups stressed the need for the media campaign to include Latino values, such as *familismo* or close family relationships, in the advertisements.[44] Advertisements were aired in Spanish on predominately Spanish-language media outlets and quit-line callers who mentioned the advertisements were eligible to receive supplies of NRT. The results showed a 57.6% increase in calls to the quit line during the media campaign. Latino respondents during the campaign were significantly younger, more often Spanish speaking, lacked insurance, and were less educated as compared with precampaign Latino study participants. Results from Latino participants showed that program completion and NRT use were similar before and during the campaign and 6-month quit rates significantly improved ($P = .04$). The researchers concluded that a media campaign targeted to reach a Spanish-language audience increased quit line reach and improved cessation outcomes among a young Latino population of low socioeconomic status (SES) in the state of Colorado. These findings may also have implications for Mexican Latina women and children who live with a smoker. Young Mexican men make up the largest demographic proportion of US immigrants,[45,46] and 39.1% of Mexican men are smokers.[47] Before the campaign, 38% of Latino callers lived with a smoker, and, during the campaign, 37.4 % of Latino callers lived with a smoker.

## POLICY CHANGE

Stein, Ellis, Savitz, Vichinsky, and Peri[48] conducted a study evaluating the prevalence rates of pregnant smokers when tobacco-control policies were being strengthened. These policies included a ban on indoor workplace smoking and an increase in the public's access to cessation treatment. The study found declines in prenatal smoking prevalence among all ethnic groups; however, African American and Puerto Rican women demonstrated the smallest decline. The investigators concluded there is a need for a greater focus on smoking cessation among pregnant African American and Puerto Rican women to reduce racial and ethnic disparities in prenatal smoking.

## FINANCIAL AND JOB STRAIN

Financial strain is associated with smoking, greater daily cigarette consumption, and smoking relapse.[49] The literature suggests that low SES smokers are as likely to attempt to quit as higher-SES smokers but less likely to be successful[50] because of the reduced access to smoking-cessation resources or other social determinants. Adverse psychosocial work characteristics may also increase the chance of poor health behaviors, such as smoking as a way to cope with adverse conditions and negative emotions.[20]

Rugulies, Scherzer, and Krause[51] examined the associations between psychological demands, decision latitude, and job strain and smoking in female hotel cleaners in Las Vegas, Nevada. Their sample included a high percentage of Hispanic women (76.2%). Findings revealed a strong effect of place of birth. Hispanic hotel cleaners who were born in the United States were 2.4 times more likely to smoke than Hispanic hotel cleaners who were born outside of the United States. This study also found that perceived low decision latitude and high job strain were associated with smoking in Hispanic hotel cleaners. Although this study did not specify whether any of the female hotel cleaners were pregnant during the study, the findings reinforce the literature that states that place of birth has a relationship to smoking and tobacco cessation.[48] In addition, some Hispanic women may work as hotel cleaners during the prenatal and postnatal periods, so providing smoking-cessation information in the workplace, particularly to Latina women who were born outside of the United States, may help raise awareness of resources to help quit smoking.

## SUMMARY

Pregnant Latina women living in the United States are a heterogeneous group represented by a variety of countries, cultures, and immigration status. Although some of the literature refers to a Latina health paradox that may serve as a protective factor against smoking for recent immigrants, acculturation may increase the vulnerability of pregnant Latina women to begin smoking. Social support treatments should be individualized to each pregnant woman based on what types of emotional, informational, or instrumental resources the woman desires. Some pregnant women are able to quit spontaneously but others need intervention.

When choosing or designing evidence-based tobacco cessation programs for use with Latina pregnant women, nurses should select programs that are tailored to embrace Latino values, such as *familismo* and *personalismo*. Second, pregnant Latina women should be given the option of receiving educational materials and other types of interventions in either English or Spanish.

Third, programs that use bilingual LHAs seem to hold promise for more-effective community-based interventions. Several studies demonstrated training models to teach lay health providers how to provide evidence-based smoking cessation programs, such as the 5 A's model or motivational interviewing, to Latino persons in community settings, and nurses could develop such training programs. The use of lay health providers may be a better model to deliver tobacco cessation treatment to a vulnerable Hispanic population that has more difficulty accessing health care. The use of financial incentives and offering tobacco cessation programs in workplaces that use a high number of Latina women, such as hotels, may be helpful. The use of financial incentives may be particularly important for Latina immigrants who are undocumented or uninsured and lack the ability to visit a health care provider or purchase resources to help them quit smoking.

The use of technology to provide social support during tobacco cessation or to educate about passive smoking risks holds promise for young Latina women, but better access to computers and other forms of technology by Hispanic persons is needed. Nurses should assess the pregnant woman's access to technology before recommending quit lines, texting, and computer-based tobacco cessation programs.

## REFERENCES

1. Cigarette smoking among adults-United States, 2006. MMWR Morb Mortal Wkly Rep 2007;56:1157–61.
2. Mackay J, Eriksen M. The tobacco atlas. Geneva (Switzerland): World Health Organization; 2002.
3. Koh HK, Massen-Short S, Elqura L. Disparities in tobacco use and lung cancer. In: Koh HK, editor. Toward the elimination of cancer disparities. New York: Springer; 2009. p. 109–35.
4. Health United States. With chart book on trends in the health of Americans. Hyattsville (MD): National Center for Health Statistics; 2006.
5. Melvn C, Gaffney C. Treating nicotine use and dependence of pregnant and parenting smokers: an update. Nicotine Tob Res 2004;6(Suppl 2):S107–24.
6. Hymowitz N, Schwab M, McNerney C, et al. Postpartum relapse to cigarette smoking in inner city women. J Natl Med Assoc 2003;95(6):461–74.
7. Matthew TJ, Rivera CC. Smoking during pregnancy-United States, 1990-2002. MMWR Morb Mortal Wkly Rep 2004;53:911–5.
8. 2001 Surgeon General's report-women and smoking: efforts to reduce tobacco use among women and girls. Atlanta (GA): Centers for Disease Control and Prevention; 2001.
9. King TK, Borrelli B, Black C, et al. Minority women and tobacco: implications for smoking cessation interventions. Ann Behav Med 1997;19(3):301–13.
10. Glasgow RE, Whitlock EP, Eakin EG, et al. A brief smoking cessation intervention for women in low-income Planned Parenthood clinics. Am J Public Health 2000; 90(5):786–9.
11. English KC, Merzel C, Moon-Howard J. Translating public health knowledge into practice: development of a lay health advisor prenatal tobacco cessation program. J Public Health Manag Pract 2010;16(3):E9–19.
12. Koh HK, Oppenheimer SC, Massin-Short SB, et al. Translating research evidence into practice to reduce health disparities: a social determinants approach. Am J Public Health 2010;100(Suppl 1):S72–80.
13. Griner D, Smith TB. Culturally adapted mental health interventions: a meta-analytic review. Psychother Theor Res Pract Train 2006;43:531–48.

14. Hispanics account for more than half of nation's growth in past decade. Pew Hispanic Center Research on Demography; 2011. p. 2. Available at: http://www.pewhispanic.org/topics. Accessed September 12, 2011.
15. Hispanic trends: a people in motion. From trends, 2005. Pew Hispanic Center; 2005. Available at: http://www.pewhispanic.org/topics. Accessed September 12, 2011.
16. Hispanic health: divergent and changing. Pew Hispanic Center Research on Demography; 2002. p. 17. Available at: http://www.pewhispanic.org/topics. Accessed September 12, 2011.
17. Statistical profiles of the Hispanic and foreign born populations in the U. S. Pew Hispanic Center Research on Demography; 2010. p. 5. Available at: http://www.pewhispanic.org/topics. Accessed September 12, 2011.
18. Dubard CA, Gizlice Z. Language spoken and differences in health status, access to care, and receipt of preventive services among US Hispanics. Am J Public Health 2008;98(11):2021–8.
19. Hunt LM, Schneider S, Comer B. Should "acculturation" be a variable in health research? A critical review of research on US Hispanics. Soc Sci Med 2004;59: 973–86.
20. Emmons KM. Health behaviors in a social context. In: Berkman LF, Kawachi I, editors. Social epidemiology. New York: Oxford University Press; 2000. p. 242–66.
21. Bethel JW, Schenker MB. Acculturation and smoking patterns among Hispanics: a review. Am J Prev Med 2005;29:143–8.
22. Fleuriet KJ. Problems in the Latina paradox: measuring social support for pregnant immigrant women from Mexico. Anthropol Med 2009;16(1):49–59.
23. Fuentes-Affleck E, Hessol N, Perez-Stable EJ. Testing the epidemiological paradox of low birth weight in Latinos. Arch Pediatr Adolesc Med 1999;153(2): 147–53.
24. Westmaas JL, Bontemps-Jones J, Bauer JE. Social support in smoking cessation: reconciling theory and evidence. Nicotine Tob Res 2010;12(7):695–707.
25. Quinn VP, Mullen PD, Ershoff DH. Women who stop smoking spontaneously prior to prenatal care and predictors of relapse before delivery. Addict Behav 1991; 16(1–2):29–40.
26. Morasco BJ, Dornelas EA, Fischer EH, et al. Spontaneous smoking cessation during pregnancy among ethnic minority women: a preliminary investigation. Addict Behav 2006;31:203–10.
27. Gaither KH, Huber LR, Thompson ME, et al. Does the use of nicotine replacement therapy during pregnancy affect pregnancy outcomes? Maternal Child Health 2009;13:497–504.
28. Swider SM. Outcome effectiveness of community health workers: an integrative literature review. Public Health Nurs 2002;19(1):11–20.
29. Rhodes SD, Foley KL, Zometa CS, et al. Lay health advisor interventions among Hispanics/Latinos: a qualitative systematic review. Am J Prev Med 2007;33(5): 418–27.
30. Campbell J, Mays MZ, Yuan NP, et al. Who are health influencers? Characterizing a sample of tobacco cessation interveners. Am J Health Behav 2007;31(2): 181–92.
31. Unequal treatment: confronting racial and ethnic disparities in healthcare. Washington, DC: Institute of Medicine; 2002.
32. Martinez-Bristow Z, Sias JJ, Urquidi UJ, et al. Tobacco cessation services through community health workers for Spanish-speaking populations. Am J Health Behav 2006;96(2):211–3.

33. Borelli B, McQuaid EL, Novake S, et al. Motivating Latino caregivers of children with asthma to quit smoking: a randomized trial. J Consult Clin Psychol 2010; 78(1):34–43.

34. Anez LM, Silva MA, Paris M, et al. Engaging Latinos through the integration of cultural values and motivational interviewing principles. Prof Psychol Res Pract 2008;39:153–9.

35. Fiore MC, Bailey WC, Cohen SJ, et al. Treating tobacco use and dependence: clinical practice guideline. Rockville (MD): U. S. Department of Health and Human Services, Public Health Service; 2000. Available at: http//www.surgeongeneral.gov/tobacco/treating_tobacco_use.pdf. Accessed September 12, 2011.

36. Prochaska JO, Velicer WF. The transtheoretical model of health behavior change. Am J Health Promot 1997;12:38–48.

37. Prochaska JO, DiClemente C. Stages and processes of self-change of smoking: toward an integrative model of change. J Consult Clin Psychol 1983;51(3): 390–5.

38. Yunzel-Butler C, Joyce T, Racine AD. Maternal smoking and the timing of WIC enrollment. Matern Child Health J 2010;14:318–31.

39. Portnoy DB, Scott-Shseldon LA, Johnson BT, et al. Computer-delivered interventions for health promotion and behavioral risk reduction: a meta-analysis of 75 randomized controlled trials, 1988-2007. Prev Med 2008;47:3–16.

40. How young Latinos communicate with friends in the digital age. Pew Hispanic Center Research on Demography; 2010. p. 5. Available at: http://www.pewhispanic.org/topics. Accessed September 12, 2011.

41. Ling PM, Glantz SA. Tobacco industry research on smoking cessation- recapturing young adults and other recent quitters. J Gen Intern Med 2004;19:419–26.

42. Munoz RF, Barrera AZ, Delucchi K, et al. International Spanish/English Internet smoking cessation trail yields 20% abstinence rates at 1 year. Nicotine Tob Res 2009;11(9):1025–34.

43. Burns EK, Levinson AH. Reaching Spanish-speaking smokers: state-level evidence of untapped potential for quit line utilization. Am J Public Health 2010;100(Suppl 1):S165–70.

44. Baezconde-Garbanati L, Garbanati JA. Tailoring tobacco control messages for Hispanic populations. Tob Control 2009;9(Suppl 1):i51.

45. Hoefer M, Rytina N, Backer B. Estimates of the unauthorized immigrant population residing in the United States. Washington, DC: Office of Immigration Statistics, Policy Directorate, U.S. Department of Homeland Security; 2007.

46. Department of Homeland Security. Yearbook of immigration statistics: 2007. Office of Immigration Statistics, U.S. Department of Homeland Security. Washington, DC; 2008.

47. Kuri-Morales PA, Gonzalez-Roldan JF, Hoy MJ, et al. Epidemiology of tobacco use in México. Salud Publica Mex 2006;48(Suppl 1):S91–8 [in Spanish].

48. Stein CR, Ellis JA, Savitz DA, et al. Decline in smoking during pregnancy in New York City, 1995-2005. Public Health Rep 2009;124:841–9.

49. Falba T, Teng H, Sindelar JL, et al. The effect of involuntary job loss on smoking intensity and relapse. Addiction 2005;100(9):1330–9.

50. Kotz D, West R. Explaining the social gradient in smoking cessation: it's not in the trying, but in the succeeding. Tob Control 2009;18(1):43–6.

51. Rugulies R, Scherzer T, Krause N. Associations between psychological demands, decision latitude, and job strain with smoking in female hotel room cleaners in Las Vegas. Int J Behav Med 2008;15:34–43.

# Gender Influences in Tobacco Use and Cessation Interventions

Joan L. Bottorff, PhD, RN, FCAHS[a],*, Rebecca Haines-Saah, PhD[b],
John L. Oliffe, PhD, RN[c], Gayl Sarbit, PhD[a]

KEYWORDS

• Gender influences • Masculinity • Femininity • Gender relations
• Smoking • Tobacco • Harm reduction

Tobacco use continues to be the leading cause of preventable death among women and men worldwide, killing nearly 6 million people each year.[1] Although the overall numbers of men who smoke worldwide continues to be substantially greater than the number of women,[2] rates of tobacco use among women are growing whereas men's rates are in decline. Women are being aggressively targeted by marketing from tobacco companies, particularly in developing nations,[2] where smoking rates remain high for both sexes[3] when compared with rates within developed countries. However, as a result of tobacco-control measures in regions such as North America, prevalence rates for both sexes have seen major declines over the past several decades, with the percentage of the population over the age of 15 years who are current smokers at 19% for men and 16% for women in Canada,[4] and 24% for men and 18% for women over 18 years old in the United States.[5] Smokers of both sexes die from tobacco use, and while some evidence indicates that sex-specific factors play a role in women's and men's morbidity and mortality rates from lung cancer, emphysema, heart attack, and stroke,[6] men's and women's tobacco-related illnesses need to be interpreted in light of the complex history of smoking-related gender influences and the shifting social norms that have shaped diversity and patterns of use.[7]

[a] Institute for Healthy Living and Chronic Disease Prevention, University of British Columbia, Okanagan Campus, 3333 University Way, Kelowna, BC, Canada V1V 1V7
[b] School of Nursing, University of British Columbia, Vancouver Campus, T201 2211 Wesbrook Mall, Vancouver, BC, Canada V6T 1V7
[c] School of Nursing, University of British Columbia, Vancouver Campus, T201 2211 Wesbrook Mall, Vancouver, BC, Canada V6T 2B5
* Corresponding author.
E-mail address: joan.bottorff@ubc.ca

Nurs Clin N Am 47 (2012) 55–70
doi:10.1016/j.cnur.2011.10.010     nursing.theclinics.com

Sex differences are biological factors that influence health and illness, amid which gender is an important social influence on health practices and illness behaviors. Although it is recognized that sex and gender interact to influence tobacco use, in this article the authors focus on gender influences and their implications for understanding tobacco use and supporting smoking cessation. Gender, defined as socially prescribed and experienced dimensions of being a "woman" or "man" in society, is evident in the diverse ways individuals embody and contextually perform behaviors.[8] Social theories of masculinity and femininity purport that when individuals engage in specific health practices, their performances reproduce or contest specific gender ideals and discourses of gender routed within broader structures of social relations.[9] As such, gender is socially constructed and reenacted in the daily activities of our lives, particularly via the practice of health behaviors.[9] For example, young men's propensity for overusing tobacco, alcohol, and drugs and their disregard for healthy eating have been interpreted as their alignment to Western masculine ideals in signifying personal strength and invulnerability to illness and disease. By contrast, caring for others, seeking professional health care, or performing self-care are practices constructed and aligned with idealized forms of femininity. Theories in gender studies, in particular the contributions of feminist theory[10–14] and critical work in masculinity studies,[15] have expanded approaches by contesting gender binaries and identifying multiple constructs of masculinities and femininities.[16] The recognition of masculinities and femininities as socially constructed and context bound has grounded gender analyses in a relational context, and has advanced a framework in which gender is no longer seen as a fixed or neutral attribute derived from biological sex[9] but as an influence that is intimately tied to social and cultural ideologies of power.

## GENDER INFLUENCES ON TOBACCO USE

Differences in smoking rates between men and women are in large part a reflection of the influence of gender and other social and contextual factors that influence tobacco use and, ultimately, interventions. Gender inequality, and the gendered roles and responsibilities assigned to women and men, influence when tobacco is used, why it is used, how it is used, and how often it is used. Though routinely taken into account by the tobacco industry to inform product development and marketing, knowledge about gender influences has not been systematically used to guide tobacco reduction and cessation strategies.[17–19]

Adolescents arguably are a subgroup of smokers for which gender influences has received the most attention. In this context, the major focus is on the social context and functions of smoking, as opposed to addiction and dependence issues. Studies using qualitative methods have addressed smoking as a marker of gender identity for adolescents, as well as the gendered meanings that teenagers, in particular young girls, attach to their tobacco use.[20–27] The gendered symbolism attached to smoking echoes the broader cultural images of what are seen as appropriate masculine and feminine behaviors, which young people draw upon to establish and communicate their identities within the social context of peer relationships.[28]

Studies using qualitative methods have also provided insights as to how gender may influence smoking during young adulthood. For example, comparative studies have shown that young women are more likely than their male counterparts to be regular daily smokers after leaving formal education and joining the labor market.[29] Other research with female smokers has suggested that young adult women use tobacco as a way to cope with the stressors connected to leaving home and establishing their own families,[30] as well as to experiences of gender discrimination they may encounter when entering the workplace.[31] Studies of gender and smoking on college campuses have also illustrated how use of tobacco and other substances is tied to cultural norms of masculinity and femininity in social and "party" contexts.[32]

Differences in smoking patterns that reflect gender influences are also evident in subpopulations. Researchers have noted, for example, significantly higher smoking prevalence rates among lesbian, gay, bisexual, and transgendered (LGBT) people compared with their heterosexual counterparts,[33–35] a health inequity that, along with higher rates of other types of substance use, is undoubtedly linked to systemic discrimination and homophobia experienced by persons who are positioned as gender and sexual minorities.[36,37] In the Unites States, the Tobacco Research Network on Disparities (TReND) has identified LGBT populations as one of several priority groups for whom interventions targeting the general population of smokers may not be effective, and for whom interventions tailored to gender are required.[38]

Within the past decade there has been considerable progress in the application of gender analyses within tobacco research, most notably in regard of research on women's tobacco use. Early influential work in the United Kingdom,[39,40] and later work by Greaves[41] in Canada, was critical to establishing the relationship between women's smoking and social disadvantage, and the need to consider how gender and socioeconomic inequalities contribute to smoking among women who are mothers. This work was fundamental to shifting the perception of women who smoke as "bad" mothers or irresponsible parents, through viewing tobacco use as tied to the pressures of parenting within the context of poverty. Before this, women who smoked were typically considered a "special population" of tobacco users, and gender-specific issues were largely neglected by the scientific community until women's health advocates forced them to the forefront of the agenda.[42] These researchers have been vocal about the potential for "unintended consequences" of tobacco-control policies on socially disadvantaged low-income women.[43,44]

Although researchers have begun to take a gendered approach to the examination of tobacco use[45–48] and tobacco policy,[49] the focus of much of the initial "gender and smoking" research was predominately on women. As an outcome of growth in the study of men's health and the influence of masculinities on men's health practices and illness behaviors, attention has been directed to the influence of gender on men's smoking and cessation. Prior to the work on health and masculinities, critical approaches to gender influences on men's smoking were virtually absent in behavioral research, aside from work addressing stereotypical representations of masculinity seen through the iconic figure of "Marlborough man" in tobacco marketing (referred to as the "cowboy factor" in tobacco marketing research).[17,50]

Recent studies of men's health behaviors indicate distinct patterns including poor self-health and risk taking, and reluctance to take up professional health care services.[51–53] The specificities of how these idealized men's health behaviors connect and collide with smoking and smoking cessation interventions are beginning to be understood. The masculinities and men's health literature, along with the authors' recent research on men's smoking in the context of their partner's pregnancy, suggests that understanding the gendered aspects of men's smoking is essential to developing effective smoking cessation interventions that are tailored to men's lives.[45–47]

In addition to the influence of gender differences shaping tobacco use, thoughtful consideration of men's and women's experiences of tobacco use also occurs in the context of gender relations within specific social contexts and settings. A gender rela-tions approach can focus on men's and women's interactions with each other and the circumstances under which they interact, to understand the way health opportunities and constraints play out.[54] Taking into account gender relations, therefore, allows for connecting masculinities and femininities, the relational positioning of intramasculinities and intrafemininities, and the relationship of these gender dynamics to the social environment and to health behaviors including tobacco use. Researchers investigating couple interactions in the context of tobacco use examined how masculinities and femininities within heterosexual couples contributed to patterns of acceptance, and resistance to tobacco reduction.[55] For example, women's constructions of their male partner's smoking have been linked to masculine and feminine ideals. Alignment with emphasized (idealized) femininity, defined as complete compliance with and accommodation of hegemonic masculinity, appeared to reinforce women's identities as supportive wives and partners, as well as their defense of men's smoking from the perspective of individual rights, and reward for the deserving good husband and father.[56] At other times, women displayed ambivalent femininities in balancing attempts to regulate men's smoking and encourage smoking cessation, with compromises to preserve men's power and need for autonomy in order to maintain relationship harmony. Research conducted in the context of pregnancy also indicated that elements of power and control reflected in relationships with intimate partners are an important part of women's smoking experiences.[57] These findings illustrate the limitations of theories and models that focus on individual choice and responsibility to explain health behaviors such as smoking and the importance of gender-specific influences.

## GENDER INFLUENCES ON SMOKING CESSATION

Gender influences have also been observed in relation to reducing and stopping smoking. In relation to cessation, women often experience less success on initial smoking cessation than men, greater negative affective response during withdrawal, and less successful cessation in relation to nicotine replacement therapy (NRT).[58–61] Research focused on smoking relapse indicates that women relapse in situations involving negative emotions (eg, conflict or stress), whereas men tend to relapse in positive situations (eg, social events).[62] The stresses of life events can also have a differing impact on smoking cessation in women and men: women are more likely than men to relapse or to fail to quit smoking because of adverse financial circumstances, whereas men are more likely to quit if they experience negative health events.[63] Experiencing pressure within social networks (spouse/family/friends) to stop smoking helps men, but not women, to reduce their smoking.[64] Researchers have also found differences in the treatment of smokers; physicians provide smoking cessation advice more often to men than to women.[65]

Although the influence of gender on cessation outcomes among young tobacco users is poorly understood,[66] some research suggests that teenage girls and young adult women are more likely to engage in cessation[67] than their male peers, and that providing gender-sensitive interventions greatly increases cessation rates.[68,69] In response to comprehensive tobacco-control measures, the prevalence of smoking among young women sees greater declines than that in young men, although an important gender difference is that young men are more likely to use more intensive approaches to cessation in the form of NRT.[70] At the same time, it has been suggested that gender influences underlies girls' vulnerability to continued smoking, because they tend to positively associate tobacco use and weight control,[71] and fears about weight changes are a barrier to cessation. As some have cautioned, the gendered issue of postcessation weight gain needs to be carefully reconsidered, as ongoing study in this domain contributes to feminine stereotypes and may work to perpetuate the myth, as originally propagated to women by the tobacco industry, that smoking "keeps you thin."[72] Of note, tobacco researchers have largely neglected the roles of masculinities and young men's body issues in cessation, and have assumed that concerns about physical appearance and attractiveness are uniquely feminine.[73,74]

## GENDER-SENSITIVE AND GENDER-SPECIFIC INTERVENTIONS

Intriguing insights about gender influences on tobacco use and cessation experiences of men and women have sporadically been taken into account in smoking cessation interventions. Interventions have tended to be generic (one size fits all), individually focused, and delinked from the many social and contextual influences that affect tobacco use. With empirical support for the role of gender influences on smoking and cessation now well established, there is a need for cessation interventions that are not only gender sensitive (ie, generic cessation programs that are tailored to address gender influences) but also gender specific (ie, programs that are designed for or explicitly targeted to either men or women from the outset). There is a small but growing body of research related to gender-sensitive and gender-specific smoking cessation interventions. A brief summary of this research follows.

### Women-Specific Smoking Cessation Research

The main focus in women-specific smoking cessation interventions has been on pregnant and postpartum women. However, the interventions designed over the past 2 decades to reduce smoking during pregnancy have not been resoundingly successful.[75–77] Interventions have included the use of individual counseling, group support, smoking cessation resources, and pharmacologic treatments. These interventions have tended to focus on individual behavior change and lessening the deleterious effects on fetal health. Prepregnancy and postpregnancy smoking cessation interventions, which focus primarily on women's health, have garnered less attention and emphasis. Individualistic approaches to treating tobacco dependence fail to address structural factors that influence smoking behavior (ie, poverty, class, age, gender, education), microsocial factors (ie, the influence of family and intimate social networks), and the effect of power inequities in the home and in workplaces. The emphasis on the pregnant woman's smoking behavior has also diverted attention from examining the effects of the partner's smoking patterns. The presence of fathers, partners, and others who smoke in the pregnant smoker's social network affect the extent of secondhand smoke exposure experienced by the woman and the fetus as well as the social climate in which efforts toward tobacco reduction occur.

A limited number of smoking cessation interventions have been designed to support women in general. In a recent systematic review, Torchalla and colleagues[78,79] examined 39 cessation studies on women smokers. Interventions with pregnant and postpartum smokers were excluded. Although there was considerable variation in treatment models, a majority of studies consisted of brief interventions, performed in North America, and focused on comparing standard treatment offered to women with an enhanced women-only treatment protocol (36 studies were performed in the United States, and 3 were conducted in Canada, New Zealand, and Sweden). For example, in some enhanced, women-specific programs, there was a focus on addressing issues such as women's weight concerns and cognitive-behavioral counseling for managing mood and stress. Although there were findings to suggest that the interventions facilitated abstinence from baseline to follow-up, the overall outcomes of the studies were inconsistent, which is to say that targeted interventions were no more or less effective than non–gender-specific programs. Despite these limitations, the investigators also note that women-specific programs help women quit smoking, and that subgroups of women seem to prefer "women-only" cessation treatment (eg, women who are mothers, who are lesbians, or who have a history of trauma). As such, they conclude that there is an imminent need to develop creative and multifaceted programs that better respond to women.

### Best-Practice Recommendations for Pregnant and Postpartum Girls and Women

Based on a systematic review of the literature, recommendations for women-centered approaches to support women's tobacco reduction have been developed.[77] These recommendations have been well received and have stimulated efforts among tobacco-control experts to revise current practices. An updated best-practice review is now available.[80] Developed primarily in the context of cessation interventions to meet the needs of women who are pregnant or parenting, best-practice guidelines that adopt a women-centered approach emphasize a woman's health as her central motivation for quitting (as opposed to focusing solely on fetal health), and in recognizing that a woman's smoking is a response to personal challenges, place "a woman's needs in the context of her life circumstances."[42] These best-practice guidelines also include the following components.

#### Tailoring

Smoking cessation interventions should be tailored to a woman's unique circumstances that affect her ability to quit. For example, pregnancy is a unique context whereby a women's readiness to quit may not correspond to the standard "stages of change" model used in most cessation programming, and whereby approaches tailored to the needs of specific subpopulations and to women's social and economic circumstances may be more appropriate.

#### Reducing stigma

This guideline is a response to the negative social responses that pregnant women encounter around their tobacco use from health care practitioners and other service providers, and how the experiences of stigma, punishment, and blame attached to social interactions around tobacco use can be detrimental to motivation for cessation. Reducing stigma may include strategies for creating empathy among service providers and designing interventions that provide women with positive and nonjudgmental support.

#### Harm reduction

This approach is one that does not require immediate, total abstinence from tobacco but that starts with addressing the needs of smokers "where they're at," working with women that smoke, assessing their readiness to change, and developing strategies that are flexible and nonjudgmental. Harm reduction includes strategies such as encouraging women to reduce the number of cigarettes smoked per day and engaging in brief periods of abstinence (eg, a 24-hour "tobacco holiday").

#### Social support

The presence of smokers in women's lives has a direct influence on a woman's cessation outcomes and her overall health. It is, therefore, important to consider patterns of smoking within a woman's social network, assess the relationship dynamics related to tobacco use, and be mindful of the influence of power dynamics between partners during pregnancy as a potentially vulnerable period in a relationship. Identifying ways to encourage tobacco reduction among partners and other family members who smoke also needs to be considered in supporting women's cessation efforts.

### Social issues integration
This approach recognizes that smoking occurs alongside other complex and intersecting social issues within women's lives, and how alcohol use and illicit substance use, experiences of violence and trauma, mental health issues, poverty, and social marginalization influence smoking and create substantial barriers to cessation, and to a woman's overall health. Efforts to address social issues include providing referrals to community supports and free cessation services for women to remove low-income status as a barrier.

These innovative and holistic recommendations for best practice address not only gender influences, but represent a fundamental shift in how smoking is addressed within the social contexts of women's (and men's) lives, beyond issues of addiction and dependence.

### Men-Specific Smoking Cessation Research

In comparison with women, there has considerably less research addressing the effectiveness of men-specific tobacco interventions. A review by Okoli and colleagues[80] uncovered only 11 research studies detailing programs that met their inclusion criteria and were targeted exclusively at men. Most of this research is from outside of North America: 45% of the studies were conducted in the United States, with the remainder originating from Australia, China, Finland, and the United Kingdom. These studies included several designs such as randomized controlled trials, cohort studies, and pre-post studies. The key findings from this review were that quit rates among men were low across the various studies, and no study specifically designed the cessation intervention to account for gender influences. For example, in a majority of studies the only men-specific aspect was that interventions were delivered to a "men-only" group. One exception in the published literature was a study of a tobacco intervention targeted to gay men that incorporated counseling and support around health issues specific this population, resulting in higher quit rates compared with the other studies that were reviewed. The results of this review highlight the need for critical attention to the influence of masculinities on men's smoking, and for increased research that examines how gender influences cessation outcomes among men.

### Cessation for Gay Men

Gay men who smoke have been the focus of a few published studies aimed at providing tobacco interventions specifically designed for this subgroup.[81] For instance, based on the encouraging findings from a pilot intervention, Harding and colleagues[81] recommended that smoking cessation programs should include discussions of alcohol and recreational drug use, mental health, sexuality, and human immunodeficiency virus, in a nonjudgmental environment that enables participants to make connections between these issues and their ability to quit smoking. Adapting cessation interventions to the culture, norms, and beliefs of gay men to address the unique circumstances surrounding their smoking has the potential to increase the acceptability of interventions for this subpopulation.

A recent survey and focus group project with gay men in Zurich, Switzerland entitled "Queer Quit" sought to uncover gay men's preferences for supports in quitting smoking that are culturally sensitive and specific.[82,83] Queer Quit study participants reported that they were likely to participate in a cessation program that was gay specific as compared with generic cessation programming, and had strong preferences for programming delivered by a community-level organization specializing in gay men's health.[83] Yet one potential barrier raised by participants was how quitting smoking might constrain their social lives within what was seen as a "smoking gay" environment.[82] This aspect speaks directly to the need for interventions that address how tobacco use is tied to social relationships, identities, and leisure practices, and may be construed as relaxing or pleasurable for persons that smoke.[84] For example, beyond an individual-level coping mechanism for dealing with stress and stigma, for some gay men smoking may also be facilitated by participation in "tobacco-friendly" venues, when there are limited opportunities to socialize in safe, community spaces that are pro-gay *and* tobacco-free.[85] Likewise, there is preliminary evidence that on occasions when gay men attempt to conceal their sexual identity, there is an increased likelihood of their smoking.[36] Panchankis and colleagues[36] hypothesize that there are pressures on gay men to fulfill masculine gender role stereotypes, and that while engaging in a masculine self-presentation or "masking effeminacy" may protect them against discrimination and harassment, it also leads to increased smoking as they cope with these gender and identity constraints.[86] However, the idea of gay-specific tailoring needs to be tempered by recognizing not all gay men will experience their identities in the same way and that there is considerable diversity within gay communities. Further intervention studies are required to determine "whether and which gay men prefer culturally adapted cessation services, and why."[82]

## PROMISING GENDER-SENSITIVE AND GENDER-SPECIFIC CESSATION INTERVENTIONS

There is a small but growing number of promising approaches to tobacco reduction and cessation interventions that take into account gender influences. Four examples are provided to illustrate innovative ways gender influences are integrated in a variety of different approaches.

### *Start Thinking About Reducing Secondhand Smoke (STARSS) Program*

Developed in 2000 in Canada by Action on Women's Addictions—Research & Education (AWARE), STARSS was designed for low-income women who are also single parents to children younger than 6 years. A unique aspect of this program is that it is grounded in harm reduction principles, and geared toward encouraging "small steps" that women can take toward reducing children's exposure to secondhand smoke if women express that they do not want to quit or are not yet ready to quit.[87] As such, the program positions itself not as a cessation program, but as a set of tools that support women to reduce children's exposure to secondhand smoke and to reduce or quit smoking only if they choose to do so. This approach offers nonjudgmental support for women who may "tune out" messages about secondhand smoke that evoke guilt and blame about the health harms of secondhand smoke for children. A key difference from other initiatives is that it intends to disrupt stigma and stereotypes about women who smoke as "bad" mothers[88,89] through a guiding philosophy that "acknowledges the love moms have for children, and...affirms the measures moms already take to protect their children in a variety of ways."[87] STARSS is not only focused on women, but on teaching health providers to address cessation in ways that are respectful, sensitive, and empowering rather than punitive or shaming.

STARSS is an example of a program that follows many of the aforementioned best-practice guidelines related to harm reduction, reducing stigma, and developing cessation programming that is women centered. Tobacco research has been explicit about the challenges that low-income women who are parents experience around cessation, as this is a subgroup that has high rates of smoking and low rates of cessation, and for whom smoking is inextricably tied to experiences of gender and socioeconomic disadvantage.[43,49] As cited previously, Hilary Graham's early work[39,40] on smoking and family health in the United Kingdom was groundbreaking in that it challenged perceptions about why mothers living in poverty smoked. Her work produced the often quoted example whereby a woman who was a lone parent explained that she would rather forgo food than cigarettes because smoking was the "only thing I do just for myself" in a context where there are few options for relaxation and dealing with the emotional and financial stressors.[39] The approach taken in STARSS also responds to the issue of the "unintended consequences" of tobacco-control policies for low-income mothers,[44,90] by recognizing that standard advice to parents who smoke to "just take it outside" might not be feasible or safe for women who are lone parents and caring for young children.[87] In this case, using a fan, or smoking near an open window or on a balcony are ways to reduce harms, rather than requiring an "all-or-nothing" approach. The STARSS program offers nurses a way to talk with mothers about smoking in gender-sensitive ways.

### Smokefree Women

Smokefree Women (SFW) is a comprehensive gender-specific and gender-sensitive program that has been created specifically to help support the immediate and long-term needs of women who are trying to quit smoking. Free, evidence-based information and professional assistance is provided through a skillfully designed Web site that connects and engages women in a variety of different ways. SFW was designed by the Tobacco Control Research Branch, Behavioral Research Program, Division of Cancer Control and Population Sciences of the National Cancer Institute.

The uniqueness of the SFW Web site (http://women.smokefree.gov) comes from their inclusion of modern technologies to attract women to the site and to keep them interested, involved, and motivated to quit smoking. Examples of SFW's innovative and interactive tools include: Teen Smokefree TXT, a free mobile service for 24/7 encouragement, advice, and tips; real-time live conversation with a National Cancer Institute smoking cessation counselor; self-quizzes with feedback on a variety of topics; computer wallpaper images to download; pledges, team challenges, and contests. The SFW team has developed videos that reveal stories of real women who are challenging themselves to live a smoke-free life, as well as emotive videos that use creative animations. In addition to streaming these videos through the SFW Web site, the SFW team has launched their own YouTube channel.

Linked to the Web site is the SFW Facebook page, established as a place where women who are trying to quit smoking or to stay quit can share stories, offer/receive tips and encouragement, and access the latest news on the benefits of living smoke free. An impressive 2500 people "like" their page! Women have access to the SFW QuitTracker that helps them track their progress during a quit, and the QuitBoost application that provides personalized encouragement messages. One woman's recent post reads: "I have stopped nicotine for 5 days, 3 hours, 48 minutes and 56 seconds (5 days). I've not smoked 155 death sticks, and saved $39.86. I've saved 12 hours and 53 minutes of my life. I like the quit counter, the more it goes up, the better I feel about myself :-)." The SFW street team attends sporting events, airports, parks, and local coffee shops, and talks to women about how smoking affects their lives. These conversations are captured in a video blog posted on the Web site. Also, the team regularly tweets short and sweet support messages on their Twitter feed.

The SFW team recognizes that the quitting process is different for every woman, and that everyone has a story to share based on their own experiences and their own reasons for quitting. The multitude of available options on the SFW Web site ensure that women have the opportunity to select the assistance that best fits their individual needs, and women in turn feel supported, optimistic, and inspired.

### Addressing Relationships that Influence Women's Smoking

Smoking cessation resources have been designed to take into account evidence related to ways that tobacco use becomes entwined in patterns of intimacy, consumption, and divisions of domestic labor in ways that influence women's efforts to reduce and stop smoking.[91] Recognizing the importance of understanding tobacco-related interaction patterns and their influence on tobacco reduction, a booklet entitled *Couples and Smoking: What You Need to Know When You Are Pregnant*[92] (available at www.facet.ubc.ca), developed as a supplement to other smoking cessation resources for pregnant women, represents an important new direction in supporting women's smoking cessation. The purpose of this resource is to provide women with: (1) information about how smoking is embedded in couple interaction patterns, (2) guidance on how to create a supportive environment for tobacco reduction within family units (eg, suggesting alternatives for the relationship functions served by smoking), and (3) strategies aimed at ameliorating experiences of stress and conflict in their relationship with their partners and in relation to broader family and social pressures that dictate "compelled tobacco reduction" during pregnancy. For example, the booklet includes vignettes describing 3 tobacco-related interaction patterns: (1) disengaged, (2) conflictual, and (3) accommodating. These patterns of interaction indicate that couples do not necessarily begin a pregnancy with a shared view of tobacco reduction, nor do they embark on cessation in a cohesive or cooperative way.[91,93] The vignettes also illustrate how pregnancy (or even plans to become pregnant) may disrupt existing tobacco-related interactions by activating a deadline for changes in the couple's identities, gender relations, and lifestyle practices.

Despite the value of increasing awareness about how relationships may change with efforts to stop smoking and create barriers to cessation, because of the potential for conflict and complex power dynamics related to tobacco use and to ensure women's safety, researchers have recommended that cessation interventions for a woman and her partner need to be delinked (ie, delivered separately).[93] A delinked approach to tobacco intervention represents a significant departure from commonly held assumptions about intervening with families (ie, as a single unit or group). This approach is supported by evidence that among pregnant/postpartum women and their partners: (1) tobacco use is a potential avenue for power and control within relationships; (2) there is potential for increased conflict associated with tobacco reduction in pregnancy; and (3) interests and motivations to change health behaviors are shaped by this microsocial context.

### Men-Friendly Smoking Cessation Support

Recognizing the challenges partner smoking poses to women's efforts to stop smoking and remain smoke free, attention has also turned to developing effective approaches to support cessation among men who smoke. Although a majority of expectant fathers who smoke want their pregnant partners to quit smoking, they are often resistant to changing their own smoking behaviors.[56] However, becoming a father is a significant transition period whereby many men's masculine ideals connecting autonomy and hedonism to smoking yield (at least in part) to protector and provider roles that are difficult to reconcile with being a dad who smokes.

Discomfort with smoking, coinciding with men's increasing interest in fathering and engagement in caring for their babies, precipitates strong desires to reduce or quit as a means to being a good role model and father.[94] Although this perceived incompatibility of smoking and fatherhood affords an important opportunity for smoking cessation, researchers report that few men were successful, and point to the lack of resources and support tailored for new fathers.[95]

Research describing fathers who smoke, factors influencing resistance to quitting, responses to tobacco-control messages targeting men, and the influence of masculinities on smoking and cessation experiences[45–47,95] is being used to inform men-centered approaches to support smoking cessation. For example, a booklet entitled *The Right Time, the Right Reasons. Dads Talk About Reducing and Quitting Smoking*[96] (available at www.facet.ubc.ca), has recently been designed.[97] Rather than a "how to quit" guide, the unique focus of this resource is on mobilizing transitions around masculine ideals to leverage behavior change when men become fathers. Men are encouraged to consider the advantages to being a dad who does not smoke and are supported in their desire to be autonomous decision makers. Masculine images and dads' self-talk are included in the booklet to strengthen the sense of peer support and reinforce a men-friendly approach. Suggestions for nurses and other health care professionals in using this booklet include: (1) starting a conversation with dads about smoking that reinforces the messages in the booklet, (2) assessing readiness to take the first step in reducing and quitting smoking, (3) supporting men in their decisions about when and how to stop smoking, (4) encouraging dads to become actively involved in the care of their infants, and (5) helping men manage the stresses associated with being a new father (eg, using exercise). Their efforts in supporting smoking cessation among expectant and new fathers has the potential to increase men's well-being, support women's efforts to reduce and quit smoking, provide smoke-free environments for their children, and strengthen family cohesiveness.

## SUMMARY

Gender is a key social determinant of health and is considered to be one of the most important influences on health behaviors including smoking. Differences in smoking rates between men and women are in large part a reflection of the influence of gender and its intersections with ethnicity, age, and social class that influence tobacco use and, ultimately, efforts to stop smoking. However, gender influences on tobacco use and cessation experiences of men and women have not been consistently taken into account in smoking cessation interventions. There is an urgent need for developing and delivering gender-sensitive (programs addressing gender) and gender-specific (programs designed for men or women) interventions in the context of tobacco dependence treatment.

## REFERENCES

1. WHO report on the global tobacco epidemic—warning about the dangers of tobacco. World Health Organization; 2011. Available at: http://www.who.int/tobacco/global_report/2011/en. Accessed August 1, 2011.
2. World Health Organization. 10 facts on gender and tobacco. Available at: www.who.int/features/factfiles/gender_tobacco/en/index.html. Accessed August 1, 2011.
3. MacKay J, Eriksen M. Tobacco atlas. Geneva (Switzerland): World Health Organization; 2002.

4. Health Canada. Canadian Tobacco Use Monitoring Survey (CTUMS) 2008. Ottawa (Ontario): Health Canada; 2010. Available at: http://www.hc-sc.gc.ca/hc-ps/tobac-tabac/research-recherche/stat/ctums-esutc_2008-eng.php. Accessed August 1, 2011.

5. Centers for Disease Control and Prevention. Vital signs: current cigarette smoking among adults aged ≥18 years—United States, 2009. MMWR Morb Mortal Wkly Rep 2010;59(35):1135–40.

6. Gender and tobacco control—a policy brief. World Health Organization; 2007. Available at: http://www.who.int/tobacco/resources/publications/general/policy_brief.pdf. Accessed August 1, 2011.

7. Curry LE, Vallone DM, Cartwright J, et al. Tobacco: an equal-opportunity killer? Tob Control 2011;20(4):251–2.

8. Johnson J, Greaves L, Repta R. Better science with sex and gender: a primer for health research. Vancouver (British Columbia): Women's Health Research Network; 2007. Available at: http://www.whrn.ca/dnload/better-science-with-sex-and-gender-a-primer.pdf. Accessed August 1, 2011.

9. Lyons AC. Maculinities, femininities, behaviour, and health. Soc Personal Psychol Compass 2009;3–4:394–412.

10. Bordo S. Unbearable weight: feminism, western culture, and the body. Berkeley (CA): University of California Press; 1993.

11. Butler J. Gender trouble. London: Routledge; 1990.

12. Butler J. Bodies that matter: on the discursive limits of 'sex'. London: Routledge; 1993.

13. Haraway DJ. Simians, cyborgs, and women: the reinvention of nature. London: Free Association Books; 1991.

14. West C, Zimmerman DH. Doing gender. Gend Soc 1987;1:125–51.

15. Connell RW. Masculinities. Cambridge (United Kingdom): Polity Press; 1995.

16. Howson S. Challenging hegemonic masculinity. London: Routledge; 2006.

17. Hafez N, Ling PM. How Philipp Morris built Marlboro into a global brand for young adults: implications for international tobacco control. Tob Control 2005;14(4):262–71.

18. Stevens P, Carlson LM, Hinman JM. An analysis of tobacco industry marketing to lesbian, gay, bisexual, and transgender (LGBT) populations: strategies for mainstream tobacco control and prevention. Health Promot Pract 2004;5(Suppl 3):129S–34S.

19. Toll BA, Ling PM. The Virginia Slims identity crisis: an inside look at tobacco industry marketing to women. Tob Control 2005;14(3):172–80.

20. Amos A, Bostock Y. Young people, smoking and gender—a qualitative exploration. Health Educ Res 2007;22(6):770–81.

21. Pavis S, Cunningham-Burley S, Amos A. Young people and smoking—exploring meaning and social context. Soc Sci Health 1996;2(4):228–43.

22. Michell L, Amos A. Girls, pecking order and smoking. Soc Sci Med 1997;44(12):1861–9.

23. Moffat BM, Johnson JL. Through the haze of cigarettes: teenage girls' stories about cigarette addiction. Qual Health Res 2001;11(5):668–81.

24. Rugkasa J, Stewart-Knox B, Sittlington J, et al. Hard boys, attractive girls: expressions of gender in young people's conversations on smoking in Northern Ireland. Health Promot Int 2003;18(4):307–14.

25. MacDonald M, Wright NE. Cigarette smoking and the disenfranchisement of adolescent girls: a discourse of resistance? Health Care Women Int 2002;23(3):281–305.

26. Seguire M, Chalmers K. Addressing the 'costs of quitting' smoking: a health promotion issue for adolescent girls in Canada. Health Promot Int 2000;15(3):227–35.
27. Haines RJ, Poland BD, Johnson JL. Becoming a 'real' smoker: cultural capital in young women's accounts of smoking and other substance use. Sociol Health Illn 2009;31(1):66–80.
28. Stjerna ML, Lauritzen SO, Tillgren P. "Social thinking" and cultural images: teenagers' notions of tobacco use. Soc Sci Med 2004;59(3):573–83.
29. Bell R, Pavis S, Amos A, et al. Continuities and changes: teenage smoking and occupational transition. J Adolesc 1999;22(5):683–94.
30. McDermott LJ, Dobson AJ, Owen N. From partying to parenthood: young women's perceptions of cigarette smoking across life transitions. Health Educ Res 2006;21(3):428–39.
31. Daykin N. Young women and smoking: towards a sociological account. Health Promot Int 1993;8(2):95–102.
32. Nichter M, Nichter M, Lloyd-Richardson EE, et al. Gendered dimensions of smoking among college students. J Adolesc Res 2006;21(3):215–43.
33. Remafedi G. Lesbian, gay, bisexual, and transgender youths: who smokes, and why? Nicotine Tob Res 2007;9:S65–71.
34. Ryan H, Wortley PM, Easton A, et al. Smoking among lesbians, gays, and bisexuals—a review of the literature. Am J Prev Med 2001;21(2):142–9.
35. Tang H, Greenwood GL, Cowling DW, et al. Cigarette smoking among lesbians, gays, and bisexuals: how serious a problem? Cancer Causes Control 2004; 15(8):797–803.
36. Pachankis JE, Westmaas JL, Dougherty LR. The influence of sexual orientation and masculinity on young men's tobacco smoking. J Consult Clin Psychol 2011;79(2):142–52.
37. Mayer KH, Bradford JB, Makadon HJ, et al. Sexual and gender minority health: what we know and what needs to be done. Am J Public Health 2008;98(6):989–95.
38. Fagan P, King G, Lawrence D, et al. Eliminating tobacco-related health disparities: directions for future research. Am J Public Health 2004;94(2):211–7.
39. Graham H. Women's smoking and family health. Soc Sci Med 1987;25(1):47–56.
40. Graham H. When life's a drag: women smoking and disadvantage. London: HMSO; 1993.
41. Greaves L. Smoke screen: women's smoking and social control. London: Scarlet University Press; 1996.
42. Greaves L, Jategaonkar N, Sanchez SE. Turning a new leaf: women, tobacco, and the future. British Columbia Centre of Excellence for Women's Health (BCCEWH) and International Network of Women Against Tobacco (INWAT). Available at: www.inwat.org www.bccewh.bc.ca. Vancouver (British Columbia): British Columbia Centre of Excellence for Women's Health; 2006. Accessed August 1, 2011.
43. Greaves L, Jategaonkar N. Tobacco policies and vulnerable girls and women: toward a framework for gender sensitive policy development. J Epidemiol Community Health 2006;60:57–65.
44. Greaves LJ, Hemsing NJ. Sex, gender, and secondhand smoke policies implications for disadvantaged women. Am J Prev Med 2009;37(2):S131–7.
45. Bottorff JL, Oliffe J, Kalaw C, et al. Men's constructions of smoking in the context of women's tobacco reduction during pregnancy and postpartum. Soc Sci Med 2006;62(12):3096–108.
46. Oliffe JL, Bottorff JL, Kelly M, et al. Analyzing participant produced photographs from an ethnographic study of fatherhood and smoking. Res Nurs Health 2008; 31(5):529–39.

47. Johnson JL, Oliffe JL, Kelly MT, et al. The readings of smoking fathers: a reception analysis of tobacco cessation images. Health Commun 2009;24(6):532–47.
48. Greaves L. Background paper on women and tobacco (1987) and update (1990). Ottawa (Canada): Health and Welfare Canada; 1990.
49. Greaves L, Barr V. Filtered policy: women and tobacco in Canada. Vancouver (Canada): British Columbia Centre of Excellence for Women's Health; 2000.
50. Krange O, Pedersen W. Return of the Marlboro man? Recreational smoking among young Norwegian adults. J Youth Stud 2001;4(2):155–74.
51. Courtenay WH. College men's health: an overview and a call to action. J Am Coll Health 1998;46(6):279–90.
52. Lee C, Owens RG. The psychology of men's health. Philadelphia: Open University Press; 2002.
53. Watson J. Male bodies: health, culture, and identity. Philadelphia: Open University Press; 2000.
54. Schofield T, Connell RW, Walker L, et al. Understanding men's health and illness: a gender-relations approach to policy, research, and practice. J Am Coll Health 2000;48(6):247–56.
55. Bottorff JL, Oliffe JL, Kelly MT, et al. Approaches to examining gender relations in health research. In: Oliffe J, Greaves L, editors. Designing and conducing gender, sex, health research. Thousand Oak (CA): Sage; 2012. p. 175–88.
56. Bottorff JL, Oliffe JL, Kelly MT, et al. Men's business, women's work: gender influences and fathers' smoking. Sociol Health Illn 2010;32(4):583–96.
57. Greaves L, Kalaw C, Bottorff JL. Case studies of power and control related to tobacco use during pregnancy. Womens Health Issues 2007;17(5):325–32.
58. Perkins KA, Donny E, Caggiula AR. Sex differences in nicotine effects and self-administration: review of human and animal evidence. Nicotine Tob Res 1999; 1(4):301–15.
59. Wetter DW, Kenford SL, Smith SS, et al. Gender differences in smoking cessation. J Consult Clin Psychol 1999;67(4):555–62.
60. Cepeda-Benito A, Reynoso JT, Erath S. Meta-analysis of the efficacy of nicotine replacement therapy for smoking cessation: differences between men and women. J Consult Clin Psychol 2004;72(4):712–22.
61. Hogle JM, Curtin JJ. Sex differences in negative affective response during nicotine withdrawal. Psychophysiology 2006;43(4):344–56.
62. Ortner R, Schindler D, Kraigher D, et al. Women addicted to nicotine. Arch Womens Ment Health 2002;4:103–9.
63. McKee SA, Maciejewski PK, Falba T, et al. Sex differences in the effects of stressful life events on changes in smoking status. Addiction 2003;98(6): 847–55.
64. Westmaas JL, Wild TC, Ferrence R. Effects of gender in social control of smoking cessation. Health Psychol 2002;21(4):368–76.
65. Young JM, Ward JE. Influence of physician and patient gender on provision of smoking cessation advice in general practice. Tob Control 1998;7(4):360–3.
66. Sussman S. Effects of sixty six adolescent tobacco use cessation trials and seventeen prospective studies of self-initiated quitting. Tob Induc Dis 2002; 1(1):35–81.
67. Paavola M, Vartiainen E, Puska P. Smoking cessation between teenage years and adulthood. Health Educ Res 2001;16(1):49–57.
68. Dino GA, Horn KA, Goldcamp J, et al. Statewide demonstration of not on tobacco: a gender-sensitive teen smoking cessation program. J Sch Nurs 2001;17(2):90–7.

69. Branstetter SA, Horn K, Dino G, et al. Beyond quitting: predictors of teen smoking cessation, reduction and acceleration following a school-based intervention. Drug Alcohol Depend 2009;99(1–3):160–8.

70. Ellis JA, Perl SB, Davis K, et al. Gender differences in smoking and cessation behaviors among young adults after implementation of local comprehensive tobacco control. Am J Public Health 2008;98(2):310–6.

71. Grogan S, Conner M, Fry G, et al. Gender differences in smoking: a longitudinal study of beliefs predicting smoking in 11-15 year olds. Psychol Health 2009; 24(3):301–16.

72. Nichter M, Nichter M, Vuckovic N, et al. Smoking as a weight-control strategy among adolescent girls and young women: a reconsideration. Med Anthropol Q 2004;18(3):305–24.

73. Grogan S, Fry G, Gough B, et al. Smoking to stay thin or giving up to save face? Young men and women talk about appearance concerns and smoking. Br J Health Psychol 2009;14:175–86.

74. Haines R, Fischer B, Rehm J. Sociocultural factors and determinants influencing smoking among youth—a literature review (Commissioned monograph). Zurich (Switzerland): Institute for Public Health and Addiction; 2007.

75. Mullen PD. How can more smoking suspension during pregnancy become life-long abstinence? Lessons learned about predictors, interventions, and gaps in our accumulated knowledge. Nicotine Tob Res 2004;6:S217–38.

76. Sarna L, Bialous SA. Why tobacco is a women's health issue. Nurs Clin North Am 2004;39(1):165.

77. Greaves L, Cormier RA, Devries K, et al. Expecting to quit: a best practices review of smoking cessation strategies for pregnant and postpartum girls and women. Vancouver (Canada): British Columbia Centre of Excellence for Women's Health; 2003. Available at: http://www.hc-sc.gc.ca/hc-ps/pubs/tobac-tabac/expecting-grossesse/index-eng.php. Accessed August 1, 2011.

78. Torchalla I, Okoli CT, Hemsing N, et al. Gender differences in smoking behaviour and cessation. J Smok Cessat 2011;6(1):9–16.

79. Torchalla I, Okoli CT, Bottorff JL, et al. Smoking cessation interventions targeted to women: a systematic review. Women Health, in press.

80. Okoli CT, Torchalla I, Oliffe JL, et al. Men's smoking cessation interventions: a brief review. J Mens Health 2011;8(2):100–8.

81. Harding R, Bensley J, Corrigan N. Targeting smoking cessation to high prevalence communities: outcomes from a pilot intervention for gay men. BMC Public Health 2004;4:43.

82. Schwappach DL. Queer Quit: gay smokers' perspectives on a culturally specific smoking cessation service. Health Expect 2009;12(4):383–95.

83. Schwappach DL. Smoking behavior, intention to quit, and preferences toward cessation programs among gay men in Zurich, Switzerland. Nicotine Tob Res 2008;10(12):1783–7.

84. Poland B, Frohlich K, Haines RJ, et al. The social context of smoking: the next frontier in tobacco control? Tob Control 2006;15(1):59–63.

85. Leibel K, Lee JGL, Goldstein AO, et al. Barring intervention? lesbian and gay bars as an underutilized venue for tobacco interventions. Nicotine Tob Res 2011;13(7): 507–11.

86. Pachankis JE. The psychological implications of concealing a stigma: a cognitive-affective-behavioral model. Psychol Bull 2007;133(2):328–45.

87. Action on Women's Addictions Research and Education (AWARE). The guide to STARSS strategies: start thinking about reducing secondhand smoke—a harm

reduction support strategy for low-income moms who smoke. Kingston (Ontario): Action on Women's Additions - Research and Education; 2007. Available at: http://www.aware.on.ca/sites/default/files/The-Guide-to-STARSS-Strategies_0.pdf. Accessed August 1, 2011.

88. Thompson L, Pearce J, Barnett JR. Moralising geographies: stigma, smoking islands and responsible subjects. Area 2007;39(4):508–17.

89. Farrimond HR, Joffe H. Pollution, peril and poverty: a British study of the stigmatization of smokers. J Community Appl Soc Psychol 2006;16(6):481–91.

90. Burgess DJ, Fu SS, van Ryn M. Potential unintended consequences of tobacco-control policies on mothers who smoke a review of the literature. Am J Prev Med 2009;37(2):S151–8.

91. Bottorff JL, Kalaw C, Johnson JL, et al. Unraveling smoking ties: how tobacco use is embedded in couple interactions. Res Nurs Health 2005;28:316–28.

92. Bottorff JL, Carey J, Poole N, et al. Couples and smoking: what you need to know when you are pregnant. Kelowna (British Columbia): British Columbia Centre of Excellence for Women's Health and the Institute for Healthy Living and Chronic Disease Prevention, University of British Columbia, Okanagan campus; 2008. Available at: http://www.facet.ubc.ca/booklet. Accessed August 1, 2011.

93. Bottorff JL, Kalaw C, Johnson JL, et al. Couple dynamics during women's tobacco reduction in pregnancy and postpartum. Nicotine Tob Res 2006;8(4): 499–509.

94. Oliffe JL, Bottorff JL, Johnson JL, et al. Fathers: locating smoking and masculinity in the postpartum. Qual Health Res 2010;20(3):330–9.

95. Bottorff JL, Radsma J, Kelly M, et al. Fathers' narratives of reducing and quitting smoking. Sociol Health Illn 2009;31(2):185–200.

96. Oliffe JL, Bottorff JL, Sarbit G. The right time. The right reasons: dads talk about reducing and quitting smoking. Kelowna (British Columbia): Institute for Healthy Living and Chronic Disease Prevention, University of British Columbia; 2010. Available at: http://www.facet.ubc.ca/Downloads/DadsQuitSmoking.pdf. Accessed August 1, 2011.

97. Oliffe JL, Bottorff JL, Sarbit G. Mobilizing masculinity to support fathers who want to be smoke free. CIHR Institute of Gender and Health Knowledge Translation Casebook, in press.

# Online Tobacco Cessation Education to Optimize Standards of Practice for Psychiatric Mental Health Nurses

Jacques (Jack) Amole, DNP, RN, PMHCNS-BC[a],*,
Janie Heath, PhD, APRN-BC[b], Thomas V. Joshua, MS[c],
Beth McLear, MS, FNP-C[d]

KEYWORDS

- Tobacco cessation • Psychiatric and substance abuse patients
- Psychiatric mental health nurses • Education • Georgia

Clinicians and researchers are concerned that individuals with a psychiatric or substance abuse disorder are experiencing a silent epidemic of morbidity related to tobacco dependence.[1,2] In 2005, the Centers for Disease Control and Prevention estimated that seriously mentally ill individuals who use tobacco products die on average 2.5 decades earlier than the general population, with the leading causes of death being heart disease, cancer, and cerebrovascular and chronic respiratory diseases.[3,4] Schroeder[5] (2004) estimated that smoking rates can be more than 80% among patients who have schizophrenia, 50% to 60% among patients with

Funding and support for this pilot study were made possible by Sigma Theta Tau Beta Omicron Chapter, GHSU Nursing Faculty Practice Group, Sharon Bennett DNP, retired faculty, Lauren Francisco MEd and Clare Billman MS, Instructional Support and Educational Design and Richard C. Woodring, D. Min, Division of Educational Design at the Georgia Health Sciences University.
[a] Department of Biobehavioral Nursing, Georgia Health Sciences University, College of Nursing, 1905 Barnett Shoals Road, Athens, GA 30605, USA
[b] Department of Biobehavioral Nursing, Georgia Health Sciences University, College of Nursing, 987 Street Sebastian Way, EC5426, Augusta, GA 30912, USA
[c] Department of Biobehavioral Nursing, Center for Nursing Research, Georgia Health Sciences University, College of Nursing, 987 Street, Sebastian Way, EC4410, Augusta, GA 30912, USA
[d] Department of Physiological & Technological Nursing, Georgia Health Sciences University, College of Nursing, 1905 Barnett Shoals Road, Athens, GA 30605, USA
* Corresponding author.
E-mail address: jamole@georgiahealth.edu

depression, 55% to 80% among those who have alcoholism, and 50% to 66% among those with another substance abuse problem.[5] Additionally, there is a significant economic burden associated with smoking-related illnesses. From 1995 to 1999, more than $75.5 billion was spent on medical treatment of individuals with tobacco dependence and an additional $81.9 billion was attributed to lost work productivity.[6,7]

Even with the staggering morbidity and mortality statistics related to tobacco use, it is reported that mental health providers fear exacerbation of psychiatric symptoms and are reluctant to help their patients quit using tobacco.[8] Although there is limited evidence to support this assumption, several studies indicated that individuals with depression who stop using tobacco products may be at a higher risk of a psychiatric relapse.[9–12] Regardless of unanswered treatment concerns, addressing tobacco use among this specialized population must be a priority for long-term health and wellness. Evidence-based guidelines have been available for 20 years to help health care providers treat tobacco dependence, yet obstacles, such as lack of training, continue to be identified by clinicians.[12,13]

Leadership from the American Psychiatric Nurses Association (APNA) recently charged psychiatric nurses to obtain knowledge and skills to significantly deter the prevalence and negative health outcomes of tobacco use.[14] Similar to studies by others, Sharp and colleagues[15] identified lack of education by nurses as a significant barrier to effectively intervene with tobacco-dependent individuals.[15–21] Attitudes and beliefs have also been identified to predict the integration of tobacco cessation interventions as a standard of care.[19,22]

Developing and disseminating an evidence-based tobacco treatment curriculum has produced successful outcomes for health care professionals to increase knowledge and confidence to effectively intervene with tobacco-dependent patients.[20,21,23] The recently developed *Psychiatry Rx for Change Curriculum* was built on the success of Hudmon and Corelli's *Rx for Change: Clinician Assisted Tobacco Cessation Curriculum*.[24–26] Although it may be argued that national efforts to target tobacco dependence with the mentally ill have been slow, initiatives to raise awareness about how psychiatric patients achieve wellness through smoking cessation have received prominent attention for action.[14,27,28]

Optimizing health and well-being for the tobacco-dependent mentally ill population may be challenging, but nurses have a long-standing history of contributing to the body of knowledge related to effective tobacco cessation interventions.[27–29] Whether it is barriers related to lack of knowledge and skills or limited professional accountability, a change in practice is needed for tobacco-dependent patients who are mentally ill.[29–31] As the APNA position statement reminds us, "failure to act on tobacco dependence equals harm."[14] Considering that the number of tobacco users would decrease by an additional 2 million individuals per year if 100,000 health care providers were to help 10% of their patients quit using tobacco products, nurses have an opportunity to learn how to overcome the devastating harm of this hidden epidemic among the mentally ill.[4]

The purpose of this article is to report outcomes from an online education program using the *Rx for Change: Clinician-Assisted Tobacco Cessation Curriculum* among psychiatric mental health clinical nurse specialists (PMHCNSs) throughout the state of Georgia. There were 3 aims for the pilot study: (1) determine attitudes and beliefs related to tobacco cessation interventions, (2) determine knowledge and self-efficacy related to tobacco cessation interventions, and (3) determine intentions to integrate tobacco cessation interventions as a standard of practice.

## METHODS
### Conceptual Framework

The conceptual framework guiding this pilot study was the Theory of Reasoned Action (TRA). Derived from the social-psychology setting, this theory was proposed by Azjen and Fishbein in 1980. The components of the TRA model are external factors (demographics, knowledge, and self-efficacy), which impact subjective beliefs (attitude toward the behavior), normative beliefs (what others think about the behavior), and control beliefs (perceived behavioral control), which impact intentions (intention to change behavior), which impact behavior (change in behavior). **Fig. 1**[32] reflects how the TRA conceptual framework was used in this pilot study.

### Pilot Study Design

A 1-group pretest-posttest design was used to determine attitudes and beliefs, knowledge, and intentions to integrate tobacco cessation interventions as a standard of practice among psychiatric nurses. After approval from the Georgia Health Sciences University (GHSU) Human Assurance Committee, the online survey was completed by the participants before and 4 weeks after the conclusion of a 1-hour Web-based education program based on the *Rx for Change: Clinician Assisted Tobacco Cessation Curriculum*. As a licensed facilitator of the curriculum, one of the authors of this pilot study (JH) has previously reported outcomes using the Rx for Change curriculum.[20,30]

### Sample

A convenience sample of 201 board certified PMHCNSs in the state of Georgia (obtained through the American Nurses Credentialing Center) received an email invitation to participate. Participants were not paid; however, 1 hour of continuing education (CE) credit was offered. Participation was voluntary, and confidentiality of responses was assured.

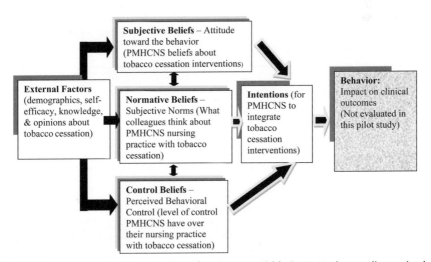

**Fig. 1.** TRA conceptual framework. (*Data from* Azjen I, Fishbein M. Understanding attitudes and predicting social change. Englewood Cliffs (NJ): Prentice Hall; 1980.)

## Instrument

The pretest-posttest instruments were a modified version of previous research reporting a Cronbach $\alpha$ of 0.95.[20,24] The underlying structure of the survey was designed to distinguish key TRA constructs that may influence intentions to integrate tobacco cessation interventions as the standard of practice among mentally ill or substance abuse populations. The pretest instrument was comprised of 51 items: 9 demographics; 15 TRA items (5 subjective beliefs, 5 normative beliefs, and 5 control beliefs); 16 self-efficacy items; 10 knowledge items; and 1 item reflecting intentions to integrate tobacco cessation interventions in practice. The format for the measurement of external factors was direct question and answers and for knowledge it was multiple-choice questions. The TRA, self-efficacy, and intention items were measured by using a 5-point Likert-type scale, with higher scores indicating a more positive response (**Table 1**).

## Education Intervention

The *Rx for Change: Clinician Assisted Tobacco Cessation Curriculum* is a turn-key training program with more than 350 PowerPoint slides that include current citations and scripted note pages, video trigger tapes, and ancillary handouts (available at http://rxforchange.ucsf.edu).[26] The full curriculum is typically offered as a 6- to 8-hour training session; however, 1-hour CE modules are available. At the time of this pilot study, the *Psychiatry Rx for Change Curriculum* was not available, thus, many of the 52 slides used for the pilot study were selected from the *Rx for Change* CE module.[26] This program is a curricular program from the University of California San Francisco School of Pharmacy and has previously reported positive outcomes to influence nursing practice by a licensed *Rx for Change* facilitator for this pilot study (JH).[19,30]

Professionals from the GHSU office of Instructional Support and Educational Design assisted with the development, implementation, and voice-over background for the online program content. The CE presentation provided a brief overview of the 5 A's framework (ask, advise, assess, assist, and arrange) and the 5 R's framework (relevance, risks, rewards, roadblocks, and repetition) for behavioral approaches to tobacco cessation intervention. The presentation also provided information on the

| Table 1 Sample questions | |
| --- | --- |
| Self-efficacy | How do you rate your overall ability to help patients stop using tobacco? (1 = poor, 5 = excellent) |
| Subjective beliefs | How valuable do you think it is to receive evidence-based tobacco cessation education? (1 = not valuable, 5 = very valuable) |
| Normative beliefs | How important do you think your PMHCNS colleagues think it is to address tobacco cessation in their clinical practice? (1 = not important, 5 = very important) |
| Control beliefs | How much influence do you think you have to help your patients become tobacco free? (1 = no influence, 5 = very much influence) |
| Intentions | What are your intentions within the next 6 weeks to give/recommend evidence-based interventions to help individuals stop using tobacco? (1 = low degree, 5 = high degree) |

*Data from* Rx for change, clinician-assisted tobacco cessation, psychiatry curriculum 2009 University of California, San Francisco (CA). Available at: http://rxforchange.ucsf.edu. Accessed June 15, 2010.

first-line Food and Drug Administration–approved medications for tobacco cessation (nicotine patch, lozenge, gum, inhaler, nasal spray, bupropion SR, and varenicline).[26]

In the spring of 2009, an invitation with an attached pretest was sent electronically to 210 prospective PMHCNS participants. During a 4-week period, 53 (25.2%) PMHCNS participants agreed to participate in the project by returning the pretest. The Web-based educational presentation was uploaded on a GHSU secure browser and released to the restricted audience of 53 participants. Four weeks were allowed for the presentation to be viewed before emailing posttests to the participants, and then the CE program was closed. Thirty (14.3%) participants reviewed the program and completed the posttest. Only participants with linked pretest and posttest data were included for evaluation. Thus, 23 pretest participants were eliminated and 30 linked participants (pretest-posttest) were included for the final data analysis.

## RESULTS

The median age of the PMHCNS participants was 56 years of age (range: 41–66 years) with the majority women (96.6%), Caucasian (96.6%), and masters prepared (86.6%). Twenty participants reported board certification through the American Nurses Credentialing Center as adult PMHCNSs, 6 as child PMHCNSs, and 1 as a family nurse practitioner. Four participants did not list a certification specialty. The range of experience in psychiatric nursing was 2 to 42 years. Of the 30 participants, 30.0% never smoked, 37.7% used tobacco experimentally, and 33.3% smoked routinely. No participants presently use tobacco products.

There were no statistically significant differences between the pretest and posttest mean scores for self-efficacy, TRA beliefs, subjective, normative, control, intentions to integrate tobacco cessation interventions, or knowledge. A 2-tailed paired t-test (significance at the .05 level) was used to analyze the data for difference (**Box 1**).

The posttest relationship between variables using the Pearson correlation coefficient analysis demonstrated a moderately strong positive relationship between self-efficacy and subjective beliefs, self-efficacy and normative beliefs, normative beliefs and control beliefs, and control beliefs and intentions to integrate. There was

---

**Box 1**
**Preintervention and postintervention subscale mean values of variables**

| Variables | Preintervention | | | Postintervention | | | Mean Difference Pretest-posttest | P Value[a] |
|---|---|---|---|---|---|---|---|---|
| | Mean | SD | Range | Mean | SD | Range | | |
| Self-efficacy | 3.57 | 0.9 | 1–5 | 3.75 | 0.82 | 1–5 | -2.69 | .467 |
| Subjective beliefs | 3.9 | 0.66 | 1–5 | 3.96 | 0.55 | 1–5 | -0.286 | .719 |
| Normative beliefs | 3.6 | 0.78 | 1–5 | 3.34 | 0.78 | 1–5 | 1.321 | .201 |
| Control beliefs | 3.26 | 0.69 | 1–5 | 3.39 | 0.62 | 1–5 | -0.631 | .461 |
| Intentions | 3.47 | 1.22 | 1–5 | 3.9 | 1.11 | 1–5 | -0.43 | .163 |
| Knowledge | 6.2 | 0.2 | 0–10 | 6.2 | 0.17 | 0–10 | 0 | [b].93 |

[a] Paired t-test significant at the .05 level (2 tailed).
[b] Wilcoxin signed rank sum test.

a weak positive relationship between self-efficacy and control beliefs and self-efficacy and intentions to integrate (**Table 2**).

## DISCUSSION

To the authors' knowledge, this is the first report of an online tobacco cessation educational program for psychiatric nurses. Although statistically significant positive outcomes have been reported by training psychiatrists and advanced practice nurses through a 2-day live course, the authors' online approach was not as robust to generate significant results.[33] In part, these outcomes were related to the small sample size and the lack of tobacco cessation content specificity for a nursing population. In addition, even though knowledge items on the survey and the educational presentation were carefully reviewed before administration, the questions may not have accurately reflected the content of the presentation. The length of time between pretest, delivery of the CE program, and posttest (4 weeks between each) was significant and may have also contributed to the small number of respondents who completed the educational program and posttest.

The results of the attitudes and beliefs among the authors' pilot study participants are similar to a study examining TRA factors to influence integrating tobacco cessation interventions among advanced practice nursing faculty.[19] The control beliefs subscale (influence to help patients become tobacco free) was the strongest relationship noted after intervention with intention to integrate scores. However, unlike Heath and Crowell's findings, the weakest relationship was normative beliefs (what others thought about intervening with tobacco-dependent patients with mental illness/substance abuse) compared with control beliefs.[19]

The outcomes from this pilot study may be useful for the development of future strategies to enhance nurses' adoption and use of evidence-based tobacco cessation protocols. Nurses are ideally suited for tobacco identification, assessment, and treatment with psychiatric and substance abuse patients. Further evaluation of online learning strategies is needed, with a larger sample size of nurses using the newly developed *Psychiatry Rx for Change Curriculum.*[25] Change in practice is related to

| Table 2 | | | | |
| --- | --- | --- | --- | --- |
| Correlation between variables after intervention (n = 30) | | | | |
| Pearson Correlation | Subjective Beliefs | Normative Beliefs | Control Beliefs | Intentions |
| Self efficacy | | | | |
| Pearson correlation | 0.548 | 0.488 | 0.381 | 0.382 |
| Significance | 0.002 | 0.008 | 0.041 | 0.040 |
| Subjective beliefs | | | | |
| Pearson correlation | — | 0.333 | 0.327 | 0.564 |
| Significance | — | 0.095 | 0.095 | 0.002 |
| Normative beliefs | | | | |
| Pearson correlation | — | — | 0.572 | 0.354 |
| Significance | — | — | 0.002 | 0.070 |
| Control beliefs | | | | |
| Pearson correlation | — | — | — | 0.577 |
| Significance | — | — | — | 0.001 |

0.002 (X2), 0.008, 0.041, 0.040, & 0.001.

empowering providers with evidence-based tobacco cessation knowledge and increasing self-efficacy to effectively intervene with the psychiatric mental health population. Numerous studies reveal the value of standardized tobacco education and the impact training has on improving clinical outcomes (helping individuals quit).[16,19–24]

## SUMMARY

The evidence is clear that tobacco dependence among patients with mental illness or substance abuse is deadly and costly. The prevalence rates for psychiatric and substance abuse patients is higher than in the general population. Considering that there is a lack of education among nurses about how to intervene with tobacco-dependent populations, the quality of care for psychiatric or substance abuse patients' is at risk. National organizations, whether nursing or other disciplines, are to be commended for initiating efforts to help eliminate the tobacco-attributable burden for patients with mental illness/substance abuse. Individually and collectively it is critical for all health professionals to transform and accelerate tobacco-control efforts through research, education, advocacy, and practice. Accessing the available *Rx for Change Curriculum* will not only help close the education gap with an evidence-based tobacco cessation program but also change practice and improve health outcomes among those with mental illness or substance abuse problems.

## REFERENCES

1. Ziedonis DM, Williams JM, Steinberg ML, et al. Addressing tobacco dependence among veterans with a psychiatric disorder: a neglected epidemic of major clinical and public health concern. In: Isaacs SL, Schroeder SA, Simon JA, editors. VA in the vanguard: building on success in smoking cessation. Washington, DC: Department of Veterans Affairs; 2005. p. 141–71.
2. Colton CW, Manderscheid RW. Congruencies in increased mortality rates, years of potential lives lost, and causes of death among public health mental clients in eight states. Prev Chronic Dis 2006;3(2):A42.
3. Centers for Disease Control and Prevention (CDC). State-specific prevalence and trends in adult cigarette smoking—United States, 1998–2007. MMWR Morb Mortal Wkly Rep 2009;58:221–6.
4. Centers for Disease Control and Prevention. Annual smoking-attributable mortality, years of potential life lost, and productivity losses—United States, 1997–2001. MMWR Morb Mortal Wkly Rep 2005;54:625–8.
5. Schroeder SA. Tobacco control in the wake of the 1998 master settlement agreement. N Engl J Med 2004;350(3):293–9.
6. National Institute of Health. State-of-the science conference statement on tobacco use: prevention, cessation and control. Ann Intern Med 2006;14:3–4.
7. WHO report on the global tobacco epidemic. Tobacco: deadly in any form or disguise. Geneva (Switzerland): World Health Organization; 2006.
8. Williams JM. Eliminating tobacco use in mental health facilities: patients' rights, public health, and policy issues. JAMA 2008;299(5):571–3.
9. Glassman AH, Covey LS, Stetner F, et al. Smoking cessation and the course of major depression: a follow-up study. Lancet 2001;357(9272):1939–42.
10. Paperwalla KN, Levin TT, Weiner J, et al. Smoking and depression. Med Clin North Am 2004;88(6):1483–94.
11. Tsoh JY, Humfleet GL, Munoz RF, et al. Development of major depression after treatment for smoking cessation. Am J Psychiatry 2000;157(3):368–74.

12. Fiore MC, Jaen RC, Baker TB, et al. Treating tobacco use and dependence: 2008 update. Rockville (MD): US Dept of Health and Human Services, Public Health Service; 2008.
13. Prochaska JJ, Hall SM, Tosh JY, et al. Treating tobacco dependence in clinically depressed smokers: effect of smoking cessation on mental health functioning. Am J Public Health 2008;3:446–8.
14. American Psychiatric Nurses Association. Smoking cessation position statement. Psychiatr Nurses 2008;98(3):192. Available at: www.apna.org. Accessed May 28, 2010.
15. Sharp DL, Blaakman SW, Cole RE, et al. Report from a national tobacco dependence survey of psychiatric nurses. J Am Psychiatr Nurses Assoc 2009;15(3): 172–81.
16. Heath J, Andrews J, Thomas S, et al. Tobacco curriculum in acute care nurse practitioner education. Am J Crit Care 2002;11(1):27–32.
17. Wewers ME, Kidd K, Armbruster D, et al. Tobacco dependence curricula in U.S. baccalaureate and graduate nursing education. Nurs Outlook 2004;52(2): 95–101.
18. Hornberger CA, Edwards LC. Survey of tobacco cessation curricula in Kansas nursing programs. Nurse Educ 2004;29(5):212–6.
19. Heath J, Crowell N. Factors influencing intentions to integrate tobacco education among advanced practice nursing faculty. J Prof Nurs 2007;23(4): 189–200.
20. Heath J, Kelley FJ, Andrews J, et al. Evaluation of a tobacco cessation curricular intervention among acute care nurse practitioner faculty members. Am J Crit Care 2007;16:284–9.
21. Kelley FJ, Heath J, Crowell N. Using the Rx for change tobacco curriculum in advanced practice nursing education. Crit Care Nurs Clin North Am 2006; 18(1):131–8.
22. Corelli RL, Kroon LA, Sakamoto L, et al. Statewide evaluation of a tobacco cessation curriculum for students in the health professions. Prev Med 2005;40(6): 888–95.
23. Prochaska JJ, Fromont SC, Leek D, et al. Evaluation of an evidence-based tobacco treatment curriculum for psychiatry residency training programs. Acad Psychiatry 2008;32:484–92.
24. Hudmon KS, Corelli RL, Chang E, et al. Development and implementation of a tobacco cessation training program for students in the health professions. J Cancer Educ 2003;18(3):142–9.
25. Rx for change, clinician-assisted tobacco cessation, psychiatry curriculum 2009 University of California, San Francisco (CA). Available at: http://rxforchange.ucsf.edu. Accessed June 15, 2010.
26. Rx for change, clinician-assisted tobacco cessation. San Francisco (CA): University of California; 2008. Available at: http://rxforchange.ucsf.edu. Accessed July 14, 2008.
27. Schroeder SA. Moving forward in smoking cessation: issues for psychiatric nurses. J Am Psychiatr Nurses Assoc 2009;15(1):68–72.
28. Rice VH, Stead LF. Nursing interventions for smoking cessation. Cochrane Database Syst Rev 2008;1:CD001188.
29. Wewers ME, Sarna L, Rice VH. Nursing research and treatment of tobacco dependence: state of the science. Nurs Res 2006;S5:S11–5.
30. Heath J, Andrews J. Using evidence-based educational strategies to increase knowledge and skills in tobacco cessation. Nurs Res 2006;55(4):44–50.

31. Sarna L, Bialous SA, Wells MJ, et al. Smoking among psychiatric nurses: does it hinder tobacco dependence treatment. J Am Psychiatr Nurses Assoc 2009; 15(1):59–67.
32. Azjen I, Fishbein M. Understanding attitudes and predicting social change. Englewood Cliffs (NJ): Prentice Hall; 1980.
33. Williams JM, Steingbert JL, Zimerman MH, et al. Training psychiatrists and advanced practice nurses to treat tobacco dependence. J Am Psychiatr Nurses Assoc 2009;15(1):50–8.

# Community-Based Participatory Research and Smoking Cessation Interventions: A Review of the Evidence

Jeannette O. Andrews, PhD, RN[a,b,*], Susan D. Newman, PhD, RN[a,b], Janie Heath, PhD, APRN-BC[c], Lovoria B. Williams, PhD, APRN-BC[c], Martha S. Tingen, PhD, APRN-BC[d]

## KEYWORDS

- Smoking cessation • Tobacco cessation
- Community-based participatory research • Action research
- Participatory research

The Public Health Service (PHS) guideline, *Treating Tobacco Use and Dependence: 2008 Update*,[1] provides recommendations for tobacco cessation interventions for smokers in clinical and health care settings. Although the number of tobacco cessation interventions delivered to marginalized populations in community settings

The authors have no financial disclosures and/or conflicts of interest to disclose.

Funding support: This publication was supported by the South Carolina Clinical & Translational Research (SCTR) Institute, with an academic home at the Medical University of South Carolina, National Institutes of Health/National Center for Research Resources (NIH/NCRR) grant number UL1 RR029882 and the National Institute of Heart Lung & Blood Institute, 5 R01HL090951-03. The contents are solely the responsibility of the authors and do not necessarily represent the official views of the NIH or NCRR.

[a] SCTR Center for Community Health Partnerships, Medical University of South Carolina, Charleston, SC 29425-1600, USA
[b] College of Nursing, Medical University of South Carolina, 99 Jonathan Lucas Street, MSC 160, Charleston, SC 29425-1600, USA
[c] College of Nursing, Georgia Health Sciences University, 987 St. Sebastian Way, EC 4511, Augusta, GA 30912, USA
[d] Child Health Discovery Institute, Georgia Prevention Institute, Medical College of Georgia, Georgia Health Sciences University, Augusta, GA 30912, USA
* Corresponding author. College of Nursing, Medical University of South Carolina, 99 Jonathan Lucas Street, MSC 160, Charleston, SC 29425-1600.
E-mail address: andrewj@musc.edu

has increased in the past decade, the effectiveness of novel community-based approaches is still unknown.[1] Over the past decade, one of these novel approaches, community-based participatory research (CBPR), has increasingly received credibility as a promising approach to address disparities in health outcomes in marginalized communities.

CBPR is a partnership approach to scientific inquiry that involves collaboration among community members, community partners, and academic researchers throughout the research process.[2] CBPR strives for maximum feasible community participation on a continuum,[3] including identifying issues to be addressed, design and delivery of interventions, evaluation of data, and dissemination of results.[4,5] Principally, as an orientation to research, CBPR can be incorporated into any research design, from descriptive studies to randomized controlled trials.[3] Compared with traditional research that is driven by academic investigators, CBPR offers the potential to improve intervention design and implementation, facilitates participant recruitment and retention, increases the quality and validity of the research, enhances the use and relevance of data, increases the rate of knowledge translation, and creates a shorter loop between research activity and community adoption of evidence-based practices.[6,7]

Despite the lauded benefits and increased use of CBPR, there are only a few systematic reviews assessing the evidence of this approach and none to date that have examined the evidence of CBPR and tobacco cessation interventions. This article reviews the relevant literature on the use, quality, and effectiveness of CBPR for smoking cessation interventions. The following research questions guided this integrative review:

1. What is the evidence that a CBPR approach improves quality of community involvement and research methodology?
2. What are the cessation outcomes of CBPR-developed smoking cessation interventions?

## METHODS

An integrative review[8] was conducted using the following databases: Pub Med, Medline (OVID), PyscINFO, and Cumulative Index of Nursing and Allied Health Literature from January 1995 to June 2011. The following search terms were used: "smoking" or "smoking cessation" or "tobacco" or "tobacco cessation" AND "community based participatory research" or "action research" or "participatory research" or "academic-community partnerships" or "institutional community partnerships." Search terms were determined after reviewing existing CBPR literature and compiling associated keywords and subject headings. Reference lists of the included studies were also searched for articles published that were not revealed in the initial search and for additional papers by the included authors for other supportive documents of the CBPR processes.

The following inclusion and exclusion criteria were used:

Inclusion criteria
1. Smoking or tobacco cessation intervention
2. Data-based studies with cessation outcomes reported
3. Community partner identified
4. Description of community-partner involvement in the planning and/or execution of research.

Exclusion criteria

1. Paper not available in English
2. Tobacco prevention studies
3. Descriptive papers only with lack of reported cessation outcomes.

## Data Collection and Analyses

Two authors (J.O.A. and S.D.N.) independently reviewed the abstracts and articles for inclusion with 100% inter-rater reliability. Data was extracted using a standardized template developed by the research team to capture all relevant data. The template was reviewed by all members of the research team and consensus reached by discussion within team members.

## Quality Scoring

The quality of the community participation and research methodology was scored using information available in the published articles. The tools used for quality scoring were originally developed by Viswanathan and colleagues[5] and adapted by Chen and colleagues.[9] The tool for quality of community participation[9] had 2 major domains: (1) nature of community involvement (selection of research questions, proposal development, financial responsibility for grant funds, study design, recruitment and retention of study participants, measurement instruments and data collection, intervention development and implementation, interpretation of findings, dissemination of findings, and application of findings to health concern identified) and (2) evidence of community-based research elements (structure or mechanism for shared decision making, study designed to remove barriers to community participation, assessed social determinants of health (SDOH), addressed SDOH through design, research team flexibility, individual capacity building, community capacity building, dissemination to participants, application to health-related intervention or policy change, and sustainability). Each item of the tool was scored as 1in (insufficient information), 1p (poor), 2 (fair), or 3 (good). Scores were summed and averaged, with possible scores ranging from 1 to 3, with higher scores indicating higher community involvement.[9]

The tool[9] to score the quality of research methodology had 9 domains: research question, study population and external validity, control/comparison group, intervention/exposure, internal validity/fidelity, primary outcome measures, statistical analyses, blinding, and funding source. Scoring for this tool was the same as the quality tool described above, with possible scores ranging from 1 to 3, with higher scores representing higher quality and research rigor.[9]

## Search Results

A total of 247 abstracts were identified from the initial review, of which 108 were duplicates and 122 did not meet the inclusion criteria, resulting in 17 papers for review. An additional hand search of reference lists with these included papers was conducted, yielding 6 additional papers, for a total of 23 papers, which described 11 cessation studies and associated CBPR partnerships.

## STUDY FINDINGS

Of the 11 studies, 8 were cessation interventions targeted to adults and 3 to adolescents/young adults (see **Table 1**). All 11 studies were developed with a marginalized community. Two studies engaged partnerships with low-socioeconomic African

**Table 1**
Summary of studies included in review

| Reference | Purpose | Community Partners | Sample/Setting | Approach/Design | Intervention | Cessation Outcomes | Quality of Community Involvement Research | Quality of Research | Comments |
|---|---|---|---|---|---|---|---|---|---|
| Andrews et al,[10] 2005 Andrews et al,[11] 2007 Andrews et al,[12] 2007[a] Andrews et al,[13] 2011 | Develop, implement, and evaluate cessation intervention in public housing Sister-to-Sister | Housing authority; Advisory CAB; Lay members | N = 103 AA women Setting: 2 public housing neighborhoods in the Southeast United States | Described partnership development Intervention development: focus groups, key informant interviews, grounded theory study, quantitative surveys Design: Quasi-experimental with 2 groups | Multilevel intervention: Community health worker 1:1 interaction weekly × 12 wk Group counseling by nurse × 6 wk Nicotine patches × 6 wk Neighborhood activities/policy CL: Written cessation materials at baseline and group attention weekly × 6 wk | 6-mo cessation 27.5% TX vs 5.7% CL (OR = 6.1–23.1) 7-d point prevalence at wk 6, 12, 24 = 49%, 39%, 39% in TX vs 15%, 7.6%, 11.5% CL Validated by CO | 2.8 | 2.6 | Met 100% recruitment goals 6-mo retention rate: 87.5% Neighborhood-level policies Randomized cluster design being conducted in 14 neighborhoods in 2 states; n = 406 women |
| Bryce et al,[29] 2009[a] | Develop, implement, and evaluate a midwifery intervention to assist pregnant women and partners to quit smoking Community Action on Tobacco for Children's Health | Local health board; midwife; steering group | N = 79 (65 women and 14 male partners) Low-SES pregnant smokers of 25 y or younger and partners Setting: Hospital maternity unit in West Scotland | Described partnerships Needs assessment conducted; training Design: Descriptive study with 1 group | Motivational interviewing by nurse midwife; Multiple modalities offered (1:1, couple, or group) NRT Home follow-up (duration of intervention not clear) | 3-mo cessation = 20.3% 12-mo cessation = 12.7% Validated by CO | 1.65 | 1.5 | 289 smokers eligible (recruitment goals unclear) 88% retention at 3 mo 47% retention at 12 mo |

| | | | | | | |
|---|---|---|---|---|---|---|
| Burton et al,[21] 2004 Shelly et al,[22] 2008[a] | Estimate the effect of a tailored multicomponent community-based smoking cessation intervention within context of state- and citywide tobacco control initiatives | Community-based organizations; CAB | N = 2537 adults in baseline interview (pretest); 1384 from original cohort completed second interview Chinese immigrants living in New York City (posttest) Setting: TX Community: Flushing, Queen, NY CO Community: Sunset Park, Brooklyn, NY | Household interviews, focus groups to prompt mobilization Design: Pretest, posttest quasi-experimental | Both communities exposed to tobacco control public policy changes over a 2-y period (October 2003 to September 2005) However, only Flushing received additional linguistically- and culturally specific community-level tobacco control interventions (public education, social marketing, posters, brochures; access to language-specific cessation resources) | From 2002 to 2006, overall smoking prevalence rate among Chinese immigrants declined from 17.7% to 13.6% (relative 23% decrease) After controlling for sociodemographic characteristics, there was an absolute 3.3% decrease in smoking prevalence attributed to policy changes with an additional absolute decline in prevalence rate of 2.8% in the intervention community relative to the CL community Self-report |

| | | |
|---|---|---|
| 2.0 | 2.4 | Citywide policies Sustainable |

(continued on next page)

**Table 1**
*(continued)*

| Reference | Purpose | Community Partners | Sample/Setting | Approach/Design | Intervention | Cessation Outcomes | Quality of Community Involvement | Quality of Research | Comments |
|---|---|---|---|---|---|---|---|---|---|
| Braun et al,[26] 2006 Braun et al,[27] 2006 Santos et al,[28] 2008[a] | Test effect of a comprehensive tobacco cessation protocol that has been institutionalized in 5 NHHCS | Imi Hale-Native Hawaiian Cancer Network representatives; community outreach workers; Department of Health; others | Clinics developed list of all smokers in past 6 mo in 5 settings; randomly selected 30 charts at each site for review Setting: 5 NHHCS | Described partnership development; Intervention development; statewide surveys, inventory of cessation services; focus groups, interviews Design: Observational | Culturally tailored Agency for Healthcare Research and Quality protocols for smoking cessation in 5 health systems Offered brief, intensive, and systems interventions based on 5 As (Ask, Advise, Assess, Assist, and Arrange) | 80%–100% of NHHCS clients asked about tobacco use 57%–100% of clients received brief intervention 21 of 50 (42%) clients completing intervention remained abstinent at 3 mo Self-report | 2.1 | 1.7 | Varying levels of adoption of intervention at 5 sites 6 y to develop protocol System changes yield likelihood of sustainability |
| Daley et al,[23] 2010[a] | Develop, implement, and evaluate pilot culturally tailored cessation intervention in urban and reservation communities All Nations Breath of Life | Native American community members | N = 108 Native American adult smokers Setting: Urban and reservation Native American communities in Kansas | Described intervention development: Focus groups; pilot testing with 4 iterations of the program; Intervention testing Design: Descriptive with 1 group | Intervention has 5 components: Group support weekly × 9 groups Individual phone counseling with motivational interviewing × 12 wk Educational curriculum Pharmacotherapy (participant choice) Participant incentives | 65% cessation at program completion 6-mo cessation = 25% Self-report | 1.8 | 1.4 | Recruitment target/ eligibility unknown No retention rates reported |

| Study | Objective | Partnership | Sample / Setting / Design | Intervention | Results | | | Recruitment / Retention |
|---|---|---|---|---|---|---|---|---|
| Froelicher et al,[14] 2010[a] Malone et al,[15] 2006 | Investigate whether tobacco industry documents in a cessation program to contextualize the social justice implications of tobacco promotion could assist AA quit smoking Protecting the Hood Against Tobacco | San Francisco African American Tobacco Free Project; and the Bayview and Hunter's Point neighborhoods | N = 60 AA smokers Setting: Public clinic adjacent to large AA neighborhood in San Francisco Intervention development included focus groups, town hall meetings, and community surveys Design: RCT | TX: 5-wk intervention program plus tailored tobacco industry and media messages (ie, to reinforce tobacco industry targeting, community empowerment, and social justice) plus phone support; NRT available CL: standard 5-wk cessation intervention, NRT available | 6-mo cessation = 13.6% TX vs 11.5 CL 12-mo cessation = 15.8 TX vs 5.3 CL Validated by salivary cotinine | 1.55 | 2.2 | Recruitment goal = 270 participants Difficulty with recruitment 37% retention at 12 mo |
| Horn et al,[24] 2005[a] Horn et al,[25] 2008 | Test an adapted American Lung Association program for American Indian Teen Cessation AINOT | Tribal partner organization, other local, state, national partners; CAB | N = 74 (54 TX and 20 CO) American Indian smokers 14–19 y old Setting: North Carolina American Indian community; 10 schools Described partnership development; Demonstrated CBPR principles throughout study Design: Quasi-experimental with 2 groups | AINOT intervention: 10 sessions, 1 h/wk, up to 4 booster sessions over 3 mo in group setting CL: Brief intervention (15-min classroom session) | 3-mo cessation: ITT 18% TX vs 10% CO) (not significant) 28.6% of men (n = 6) in TX vs 14.3% (n = 1) of men in CL reported cessation; no women reported cessation Self-report | 3 | 2.3 | Recruitment goal = 200 youths Challenge to recruit expected sample in time frame 58% retention rates |

(continued on next page)

**Table 1**
*(continued)*

| Reference | Purpose | Community Partners | Sample/Setting | Approach/Design | Intervention | Cessation Outcomes | Quality of Community Involvement | Quality of Research | Comments |
|---|---|---|---|---|---|---|---|---|---|
| Ma et al,[16] 2004 Ma et al,[17] 2005 Ma et al,[18] 2006 Wu et al,[19] 2009[a] | Develop and test culturally tailored smoking cessation for Chinese American smokers | Asian Tobacco Education and Cancer Awareness Research Special Population Network; Asian Community Health Coalition | N = 122 Asian American smokers Setting: New York City | Described partnership formation Feasibility testing Comprehensive CBPR model Design: Experimental; pretest and posttest design with 2 groups | TX: 4 individualized counselor-led motivational interviewing sessions and NRT CL: 4 health education groups | 6-mo cessation 67% TX vs 32% CL Validated by CO | 3.0 | 2.7 | Met recruitment goals 88% retention at 6 mo Planning larger RCT |
| McDonnell et al,[20] 2011[a] | Develop, implement, and evaluate online cessation program tailored for Korean Americans Quitting is Winning | Korean CAB in California | N = 1112 Korean American smokers; 88% men Setting: Recruited via advertisements in major newspapers and Web sites in the Korean American community in the United States | Described partnership formation Conducted in-depth interviews Intervention development Design: RCT | TX: Online self-help based on Stop Smoking Center program; cognitive behavioral self-help program based on stages of change with 6 sections CL: mailed booklet version of online program Both materials translated into Korean | At 50 wk, no difference in 30-day cessation between the Internet group (11%) vs booklet (13%) Quitting was higher among participants in intervention group who completed the online program (26% vs 10%) who did not complete Self-report | 1.7 | 2.6 | 2.5-y recruitment period 48% completed assessments in TX and 57% in CL |

| Study | Objective | Partners | Sample/Setting | Methods | Intervention | Outcomes | | | Sustainability |
|---|---|---|---|---|---|---|---|---|---|
| Mendenhall et al,[31] 2008 Mendenhall et al,[32] 2010[a] | Develop, implement, and test an intervention that engages local media and providers to reduce on-campus smoking at Job Corp Students Against Nicotine and Tobacco Addition | Students, teachers, and administrators in Minneapolis/St Paul Job Corps | 200–250 students on campus on average, with 6- to 18-mo residency; 40% smoke Setting: Job Corp Campus in Minneapolis/St Paul | Described partnership development; Intervention development: surveys, focus groups; implementation of system-wide changes Design: Cross-sectional with prevalence surveys every 3 mo | Several system-wide changes on campus involving 1. Fighting stress and boredom (alternative activities) 2. Changing physical environment 3. Changing policies 4. Revising smoking cessation education and support | No change in overall smoking prevalence on campus Increasing number of students report smoking less cigarettes per day ($P<.018$) Self-report | 2.4 | 1.5 | Policy changes Sustainable beyond grant funding |
| Woodruff et al,[30] 2007[a] | Test Internet-based teen cessation intervention Breathing Room Study | School partners | N = 136 teen smokers Setting: 14 high schools randomized to TX or CL in San Diego county | Partnership development Contributions to recruitment, study design, and materials Design: Randomized cluster design (7 schools per condition); analyses by individuals | TX: Seven 45-min Internet-based, virtual reality world combined with motivational interviewing over a 7-wk period CL: Measurement only | TX participants were more likely to report abstinence during past week immediately after intervention (35% vs 22% $P<.01$), yet no differences at 12 mo (38% vs 29%) Only number of times quit was significant at 12 mo (2.4 vs 1.7, $P<.05$) Self-report | 2.4 | 2.5 | Target recruitment unknown; 300 students showed interest, 200 eligible 73% retained |

*Abbreviations:* AA, African American; AINOT, American Indian Not On Tobacco; CAB, community advisory board; CL, control; CO, comparison; ITT, intent to treat; NHHCS, Native Hawaiian Health Care Systems; NRT, nicotine replacement therapy; OR, odds ratio; RCT, randomized controlled trial; SES, socioeconomic status; TX, Treatment.

[a] Major paper.

American communities,[10–15] 3 with Asian communities,[16–22] 2 with American Indian communities,[23–25] and 1 with a Native Hawaiian community.[26–28]

Several studies used a CBPR approach to socioculturally tailor the PHS guidelines for individuals using both behavioral counseling and pharmacotherapeutics.[10–19,23,29] Shelley and colleagues[21,22] evaluated the effect of community-wide policy changes on cessation, in addition to a cadre of PHS-based cessation programs and resources in the treatment community. Froelicher and colleagues[14,15] enhanced their 5-week PHS-guided intervention (ie, counseling and nicotine replacement therapy [NRT]) with tailored tobacco industry and media messages to reinforce tobacco industry targeting the African American community. Santos and colleagues[26–28] implemented PHS recommendations for system-level changes (ie, 5 As: Ask, Advise, Assess, Assist, and Arrange) in 5 health systems. Two studies used a CBPR approach to develop an Internet-based cessation intervention: one for teens in school systems[30] and the other, a tailored Internet-based cessation, for a national sample of Korean Americans.[20]

*Research question 1: What is the evidence that a CBPR approach improves quality of community involvement and research methodology?*

Based on the inclusion criteria, all studies included academic or clinical investigators and community partners. Furthermore, an advisory board or a steering committee guided all intervention studies. Several studies showed that the original question and need for the tobacco cessation intervention originated from the community.[10–15,20,23–25,31,32] In other studies, the origin was either unknown and/or the academic or community partner. The partnerships were used to conduct needs assessment surveys (quantitative and/or qualitative),[10–15,21,22,29,31,32] intervention development,[10–23,26–28,30–32] recruitment of participants,[10–28,30–32] intervention delivery,[10–19,21–28,31,32] evaluation,[10–13,16–19,24–28,31,32] and dissemination.[10–13,16–19,24,25,31,32]

The quality of community involvement varied, with quality scores ranging from 1.5 to 3 (the highest score possible was 3). Those with lower community involvement scores had challenges with participant recruitment and retention.[14,15,29] An exception was the study conducted by Horn and colleagues[24,25] that tested a cessation intervention for Native American teens in school settings and demonstrated high community involvement throughout the process (scored 3/3), yet only recruited 39% of the intended sample.

The studies with higher community scores were more likely to involve the community with dissemination.[10–13,16–19,24,25,31,32] Dissemination in community settings was typically town hall forums or community meetings or workshops, advisory or steering groups, newsletters, and local media. Several studies implemented policy changes in the targeted setting,[10–13,21,22,26–28,31,32] which potentially may increase the likelihood of sustainability. Two studies[24,25,31,32] described sustainability of the intervention after initial grant funding because of leadership, systems and/or environmental changes, and governing infrastructures.

The quality of the research methodology varied, with quality scores ranging from 1.4 to 2.7. The 7 studies with quasi-experimental or experimental designs[10–22,24,25,30] scored 2.2 or higher. The remaining 4 studies were descriptive or observational studies with 1 group only.[21–23,29,31,32] Eight studies measured abstinence rates at 6 months or longer[10–23,29,30]; yet 4 of these 8 studies[20–23,30] did not biochemically validate self-report outcomes.

*Research question 2: What are the cessation outcomes of CBPR-developed smoking cessation interventions?*

As shown in **Table 1**, the cessation outcomes varied by study design, intervention dosages and intensity, intervention content and delivery, study goals, resources, and duration. The 2 studies that scored 2.5 or higher quality scores for both quality in community involvement and research rigor demonstrated significant treatment outcomes for the 6-month cessation compared with the control condition. For example, Wu and colleagues[16–19] partnered with the Asian Community Health Coalition in New York City, which was part of the larger Asian Tobacco Education and Cancer Awareness Research Special Population Network.[18] A series of formative studies were conducted, with the team revising the study design and implementation over time, leading to the development of an intervention with tailored motivational interviewing counseling sessions, packet of self-help materials, and NRT. The investigators worked with the coalition and community members to tailor the intervention to meet the cultural and linguistic needs of the Chinese American community. The 7-day point prevalence abstinence rate at 6 months was 67% in the treatment condition compared with 32% in the control condition.[19]

Similarly, Andrews and colleagues[10–13] partnered with public housing officials and residents to develop a multilevel cessation intervention for African American women (ie, *Sister-to-Sister*) in public housing neighborhoods. The original interest for the intervention was generated by a community partner, and over time, the partners developed an intervention with 4 major components: neighborhood-level component (2 anti-smoking activities and 1 policy change), peer groups (behavioral counseling), 1:1 coaching sessions by community health workers, and NRT. The 7-day point prevalence abstinence rate at 6 months was 39% in the treatment condition compared with 11.5% in the control condition.[12] Both these studies adapted the PHS guideline recommendations for the engaged community and incorporated the local context of the community to develop and implement the intervention. Both these studies were considered pilot studies for larger randomized trials, and based on these pilot data, the *sister-to-sister* intervention is at present being tested in a larger trial in 16 neighborhoods (National Institutes of Health grant number 5 R01HL090951-03, PI: J. Andrews).

## DISCUSSION

This review highlights several strengths of using a CBPR approach and engaging with communities to develop, implement, and evaluate smoking cessation interventions. A CBPR approach can be used by interprofessional academicians and diverse community partners to develop smoking cessation interventions with marginalized communities. CBPR can be effective in enhancing community input, building community capacity, and addressing barriers to health in study participants who have historically been underrepresented in research.[33] A CBPR approach with high levels of community involvement, as highlighted in this review, has been used successfully to partner with communities to conduct needs assessment surveys, develop interventions, recruit participants, and deliver, evaluate, and disseminate interventions. All studies included in this review had evidence of a community advisory or steering board to guide the processes of the research.

Another strength highlighted in this review is that CBPR assists with the external validity challenges of traditional translational research or translating specific findings from highly controlled trials to real-world community interventions.[4] Most studies in this review based their cessation interventions on the PHS guideline recommendations, yet delivered these evidence-based modalities within diverse contexts, and situated the intervention within cultural, environmental, and community factors. The academic partners contributed expertise on the PHS guideline and evidence-based approaches to cessation, whereas the community partners contributed expertise on the local context applicable to the community. Furthermore, as suggested by others,[34] the complexity of interactions between the structure, processes, and goals of the intervention and those of the community itself arises from and is strengthened by the knowledge of the community. This unique type of partnership, blend of expertise, and knowledge generation help to transcend some of these challenges in translating evidence-based interventions into complex community settings.[2,33]

One of the major goals of CBPR is to enhance collective action for change,[1] and several papers demonstrated evidence of system-level and/or policy changes in the engaged community practice or community setting. System-level and policy changes are more likely to be sustained over time, as compared with traditional research that often ends once grant funding is over. The involvement and mobilization of community members from the onset, and working through the complexities of institutionalization and sustainability of a health-promoting intervention, are likely to foster community empowerment and social action over time.[35–38] Ideally, empowerment is both a process and an outcome of CBPR.[39]

Besides highlighting strengths, this review also highlights several challenges of using CBPR. In practice, CBPR is used in varying degrees of the established principles of "ideal CBPR" frequently reported by Israel and colleagues.[2] For example, one of the major principles of CBPR is that the community is involved with all phases of the research process. However, there was evidence that the original research question was derived from the community in only 6 of the 11 studies. Less than half of the studies documented the community's involvement with dissemination and even fewer discussed plans for sustainability of the intervention. As others report,[38] adherence to the ideal CBPR model is very challenging for these partnerships. The process of defining the community itself can be complex, whether it may be from a geographically defined community that may be too small to adequately recruit participants for a clinical trial or from a community that is diffuse and larger with which establishing meaningful and representative partnerships is difficult.[38]

Another challenge highlighted by the Froelicher study[14,15] in this review and others in the literature[3,38,40] is the navigation of the institutional review board (IRB) process for community-based studies. Navigating the IRB for CBPR studies is often time consuming. Either a lack of understanding or the differing interpretations of the institutional and federal IRB regulations by the IRB administrators and investigators may impede the process. There remains controversy about the appropriate criteria for evaluating CBPR proposals and the associated ethical implications.[3] Until these controversies are resolved and consensus is reached, this area will likely remain a challenge for CBPR partnerships.

The time involved in developing relationships, building trust, and sustaining intervention effects is another frequently documented challenge in the conduct of CBPR.[2,4,6,7,36,39] As noted in this review, partnerships may take several years to develop. The development and feasibility testing of interventions takes considerable time with these unique partnerships, which then is compounded with the challenges to sustain grant funding or other financial resources over many years. Several partnerships in this review had weathered this process and demonstrated a 10-year or longer relationship.[10–13,16–19] However, the time factor can be problematic on many fronts, especially for the junior investigator attempting promotion and tenure status, changes in leadership in both the academic and community settings, and other transitions and unforeseen obstacles that may occur.[13,38] This can be especially difficult in marginalized communities where both residents and the involved partnering organizations may be transitory.[13]

This review highlights the challenge of maintaining the rigor of academic-preferred research designs (ie, randomized controlled trials) and the dance of incorporating community preferences, which typically do not involve research, but rather services and programs in the community.[4,36,38] Seven of the 11 studies incorporated a quasi-experimental or an experimental design, yet only 3 of these 7 met other commonly accepted cessation treatment outcome criteria of reporting at least 6-month abstinence rates that are biochemically verified.[41,42] Increasingly, investigators support the practice that experimental designs may not always be feasible or appropriate to adequately test the effectiveness of community-based interventions.[3,34] For example, observational studies, as used by 4 of the included studies in this review, are becoming increasingly recognized as a practical and ethical alternative to randomized controlled trials that allows for strong causal inference.[34,43,44]

Community interventions are complex interactions, expensive, and labor intensive. Although this review did not assess the funding level for these partnerships and intervention studies, CBPR-developed interventions are often unfunded or underfunded because of the complexities in which they are administered and within the prevailing political, social, and environmental interactions in which they occur.[34] Several partnerships and studies included in this review discussed the challenges of not only sustaining the partnership but also funding over time to continue and sustain the cessation intervention.[13,24,25,31,32]

Besides strengths and challenges, this review also highlights the need for additional research. For example, several studies highlighted contributors to success in their partnership, such as champions and leaders at multiple levels within the community and the engaged organizations who continue to facilitate the work and keep the partnerships mobilized.[13,16-18,24,25] Shared decision making, communication processes, and mutual interest in the intervention are also frequently mentioned.[13,24,25,31,32] These variables and others have been recently described in the literature as CBPR partnership readiness indicators.[45,46] Although the concept of CBPR partnership readiness and related tools is emerging, additional research is needed to better understand how and why some partnerships are effective and others are not, as well as an improved understanding of the levels of readiness and how to leverage partnership readiness (ie, from partnership initiation to social action and policy change) for CBPR partners and their interventions.

Of the 11 studies included in this review, the 2 scoring highest in community involvement and research quality demonstrated promise for effective cessation outcomes using this approach.[10-13,16-19] However, both these studies were conducted with limited number of participants (ie, 103–111 participants) and were pilot studies for larger randomized trials. The ability to sustain the partnerships, sustain the effects of the interventions, and promote policy and social action are important aspects of CBPR to be achieved; yet little evidence exists on how to accomplish this. Furthermore, the question is the possibility of scaling up a CBPR-developed cessation intervention shown to be effective in one community to other heterogeneous communities for a randomized controlled trial. If the intervention is replicated in other communities, the additional CBPR processes need to be undertaken with the new communities to facilitate the buy-in, ownership, and adoption of the intervention are unclear. Further research will be needed to understand and guide best practices for these processes.

Finally, it is difficult to truly assess the CBPR effect of cessation interventions. Cessation intervention studies conducted with marginalized communities, regardless of the CBPR or traditional approach, often vary in content, delivery, duration, and study design, making comparisons of outcomes a challenge.[47] As Buchanan and colleagues[3] noted, to adequately test the CBPR effect, the ideal research design would be a cluster randomized trial that compares communities randomized to the CBPR process with a comparison condition of a traditional researcher-initiated investigation. This type of investigation, however, would be extremely complex and likely not practical.[3]

There are several potential limitations of this review. The data compiled for this review, including quality scores, were derived from the available published literature only. CBPR processes may not have been described in detail because of restrictions in publications (ie, page limits). Furthermore, the search strategy identified only articles published in peer-reviewed journals, and other dissemination materials from authors may have been excluded.

## SUMMARY

Although the quality of community involvement and research rigor varies, a well-designed CBPR approach is showing promise in working with marginalized and hard-to-reach communities to promote cessation outcomes. A CBPR approach provides strengths in overcoming challenges in translating evidence into real-world settings, contextualizing the intervention, and sustaining long-term behavior change. Challenges such as time requirements, complexities of the partnership and processes, IRB procedures, maintaining research rigor, and scaling-up CBPR efforts to adequately test effects of interventions exist. This review provides a baseline of evaluation for current efforts of CBPR-developed smoking cessation interventions and recommendations to guide future intervention development and evaluation efforts.

## REFERENCES

1. Fiore MC, Jaén CR, Baker TB, et al. Treating tobacco use and dependence: 2008 update. Clinical practice guideline. Rockville (MD): U.S. Department of Health and Human Services. Public Health Service; 2008.
2. Israel B, Schulz A, Parker E. Review of community-based research: addressing partnership approaches to improve public health. Annu Rev Public Health 1998;19:173–202.
3. Buchanan DR, Miller F, Wallerstein N. Ethical issues in community-based participatory research: balancing rigorous research with community participation in community intervention studies. Prog Community Health Partnersh 2007;1:153–60.
4. Wallerstein N, Duran B. Conceptual historical and practice roots of community-based participatory research and related participatory traditions. In: Minkler M, Wallerstein N, editors. Community-based participatory research for health. Indianapolis (IN): Jossey-Bass; 2003. p. 27–52.
5. Viswanathan M, Ammerman A, Eng E, et al. Community-based participatory research: assessing the evidence. Evidence Report/Technology Assessment No. 99 (Prepared by RTI–University of North Carolina Evidence-Based Practice Center under Contract No. 290-02-0016). AHRQ Publication 04-E022-2. Rockville (MD): Agency for Healthcare Research and Quality; 2004.
6. Lantz PM, Viruell-Fuentes E, Israel BA, et al. Can communities and academia work together on public health research? Evaluation results from a community-based participatory research partnership in Detroit. J Urban Health 2001;78: 495–507.
7. Minkler M. Community-based participatory research. 2008. Available at: http://obssr.od.nih.gov/scientific_areas/methodology/community_based_participatory_research/index.aspx. Accessed January 5, 2011.
8. Whittemore R, Knafl K. The integrative review: updated methodology. J Adv Nurs 2005;52:546–53.

9. Chen PG, Diaz N, Lucas G, et al. Dissemination of results in community based participatory research. Am J Prev Med 2010;39:372–8.
10. Andrews JO, Felton G, Wewers ME, et al. Sister to Sister: a pilot study to assist African American women in subsidized housing to quit smoking. South Online J Nurs Res 2005;1:2–23.
11. Andrews J, Bentley G, Crawford S, et al. Using community-based participatory research to develop a culturally sensitive smoking cessation intervention with public housing neighborhoods. Ethn Dis 2007;17:331–7.
12. Andrews JO, Felton F, Wewers ME, et al. The effect of a multi-component smoking cessation intervention in African American women residing in public housing. Res Nurs Health 2007;30:45–60.
13. Andrews JO, Tingen MS, Jarriell S, et al. Application of a CBPR framework to inform a multi-level smoking cessation intervention in public housing neighborhoods. Am J Community Psychol, in press.
14. Froelicher ES, Doolan D, Yerger VB, et al. Combining community participatory research with a randomized clinical trial: the Protecting the Hood Against Tobacco (PHAT) smoking cessation study. Heart Lung 2010;39:50–63.
15. Malone RE, Yerger VB, McGruder C, et al. "It's like Tuskegee in reverse": a case study of ethical tensions in institutional review board review of community-based participatory research. Am J Public Health 2006;96:1914–9.
16. Ma GX, Toubbeh JI, Su X, et al. ATECAR: an Asian American community-based participatory research model on tobacco and cancer control. Health Promot Pract 2004;5:382–94.
17. Ma GX, Fang C, Shive S, et al. A culturally enhanced smoking cessation study among Chinese and Korean smokers. Int Electron J Health Educ 2005;8:1–10.
18. Ma GX, Tan Y, Toubbeh JI, et al. Asian Tobacco Education and Cancer Awareness Research Special Population Network. Cancer 2006;107:1995–2005.
19. Wu D, Ma GX, Zhou K, et al. The effect of a culturally tailored smoking cessation for Chinese American smokers. Nicotine Tob Res 2009;11:1448–57.
20. McDonnell D, Kazinets G, Lee H, et al. An Internet-based smoking cessation program for Korean Americans: results from a randomized controlled trial. Nicotine Tob Res 2011;13:336–43.
21. Burton D, Fahs M, Chang JL, et al. Community-based participatory research on smoking cessation among Chinese Americans in Flushing, Queens, New York City. J Interprof Care 2004;18:443–5.
22. Shelley D, Fahs M, Yerneni R, et al. Effectiveness of tobacco control among Chinese Americans: a comparative analysis of policy approaches versus community-based programs. Prev Med 2008;47:530–6.
23. Daley CM, Greiner KA, Nazir N, et al. All nations breath of life: using community-based participatory research to address health disparities in cigarette smoking among American Indians. Ethn Dis 2010;20:334–8.
24. Horn K, McGloin T, Dino G, et al. Quit and reduction rates for a pilot study of the American Indian Not On Tobacco (N-O-T) program. Prev Chronic Dis 2005;2:A13.
25. Horn K, McCracken L, Dino G, et al. Applying community-based participatory research principles to the development of a smoking-cessation program for American Indian teens: "telling our story". Health Educ Behav 2008;35:44–69.
26. Braun KL, Tsark J, Santos LA, et al. 'Imi Hale—the Native Hawaiian cancer awareness, research, and training network: second-year status report. Asian Am Pac Isl J Health 2003;10:4–16.
27. Braun K, Tsark J, Santos L, et al. Building Native Hawaiian capacity in cancer research and programming: the legacy of 'Imi Hale. Cancer 2006;107(Suppl 8):2082–90.

28. Santos L, Braun KL, Ae'a K, et al. Institutionalizing a comprehensive tobacco-cessation protocol in an indigenous health system: lessons learned. Prog Community Health Partnersh 2008;2:279–89.

29. Bryce A, Butler C, Gnich W, et al. CATCH: development of a home-based midwifery intervention to support young pregnant smokers to quit. Midwifery 2009;25:473–82.

30. Woodruff SI, Conway TL, Edwards CC, et al. Evaluation of an Internet virtual world chat room for adolescent smoking cessation. Addict Behav 2007;32:1769–86.

31. Mendenhall R, Whipple H, Harper P, et al. Students against nicotine and tobacco addiction (SANTA): community-based participatory research in a high-risk young adult population. Fam Syst Health 2008;26:225–31.

32. Mendenhall T, Harper P, Stephenson H, et al. The SANTA project. Community-based prevention marketing: organizing a community for health behavior intervention. Health Promot Pract 2007;8:154–63.

33. Horowitz CR, Robinson M, Seifer S. Community-based participatory research from the margin to the mainstream: are researchers prepared? Circulation 2009;119:2633–42.

34. Trickett EJ, Beehler S, Deutsch C, et al. Advancing the science of community level interventions. Am J Public Health 2011;101:1410–9.

35. Freire P. Pedagogy of the oppressed. New York: Continuum; 2007 (first published in Portuguese, 1968; first English translation, 1970).

36. Minkler M. Community-based research partnerships: challenges and opportunities. J Urban Health 2005;82(Suppl 2):3–12.

37. Wallerstein N, Duran B. Community-based participatory research contributions to intervention research the intersection of science and practice to improve health equity. Am J Public Health 2010;100(Suppl 1):S40–6.

38. Blumenthal D. Is community-based participatory research possible? Am J Prev Med 2011;40:386–9.

39. Clinical and Translational Science Awards, Community Engagement Key Function Committee. Principles of community engagement. 2nd edition. Washington, DC: US Government Printing Office; 2011. NIH Publication No. 11-7782.

40. Wolf L. The research ethics committee is not the enemy: oversight of community-based participatory research. J Empir Res Hum Res Ethics 2010;5:77–86.

41. Williams GC, Borrelli B, Jordan PJ, et al. Measuring tobacco dependence treatment outcomes: a perspective from the behavior change consortium. Ann Behav Med 2005;29:11–9.

42. Hughes JR, Keely JP, Niaura RS, et al. Measures of abstinence in clinical trials: issues and recommendations. Nicotine Tob Res 2004;5:13–25.

43. West S, Duan N, Pequegnat W, et al. Alternatives to the randomized controlled trial. Am J Public Health 2008;98:1359–66.

44. Shadish WR, Cook TD, Campbell DT. Experimental and quasi-experimental designs for generalized causal inference. Boston: Houghton Mifflin; 2002.

45. Andrews JO, Cox ME, Newman SD, et al. Development and evaluation of a toolkit to assess partnership readiness for community-based participatory research. Prog Community Health Partnersh 2011;5:183–8.

46. Andrews JO, Meadows O, Newman S, et al. Partnership readiness to conduct CBPR. Health Educ Res 2010. [Epub ahead of print].

47. Cox LS, Okuyemi K, Choi WS, et al. A review of tobacco use treatments in US ethnic minority populations. Am J Health Promot 2011;25:S11–30.

# Tobacco Quitlines in the United States

Elizabeth E. Fildes, EdD, RN, CNE, CARN-AP[a,b,*],
Marta A.T. Wilson, MS, MFT, CPC, LCADC, NCC, DCC[c],
Betty Jo Crawford, RN, BSN[d], Salome Kapella-Mshigeni, MPA, MPH[d],
Lisa A. Wilson, BS, MEd, CRCP[e], Wallace Henkelman, EdD, RN[a]

KEYWORDS

• Tobacco use • Quitlines • Helpline • Group therapy

## TOBACCO USE AND TRENDS IN THE UNITED STATES

Tobacco use is the number one preventable cause of death and disability in the United States today.[1] More Americans are killed annually by smoking than alcohol use, motor vehicle accidents, AIDS, homicide, suicide, fires, and drugs combined.[2] In 2010, the Centers for Disease Control and Prevention (CDC) reported that 19.3% of adults aged 18 years and older reported being smokers.[3] Despite a decrease in prevalence rates, 1 in 5 adult Americans continue to smoke.[3]

### The Role of Quitlines in the Comprehensive Tobacco Control Program

The CDC has prepared best practices[4] to support each state's efforts to organize their tobacco control program into an integrated and effective structure. To decrease the

Funding Sources for the Nevada Tobacco Users' Helpline: This research project was made possible through 2 funding sources: Nevada State Health Division and Southern Nevada Health District, from the Centers for Disease Control and Prevention.
Disclosure: This publication article was supported by the Nevada State Health Division through Grant Number 5U58DP002003-03 from Centers for Disease Control and Prevention. Its contents are solely the responsibility of the authors and do not necessarily represent the official views of the Nevada State Health Division nor Centers for Disease Control and Prevention.
Disclaimer: Article is for educational purposes, not to be considered medical advice.
[a] School of Nursing, Touro University Nevada, 854 American Pacific Drive, Henderson, NV 89104, USA
[b] Department of Psychiatry, University of Nevada School of Medicine, 6375 West Charleston Boulevard, Suite A-172, Las Vegas, NV 89146, USA
[c] Division of Counseling and Prevention, Department of Psychiatry, University of Nevada School of Medicine, 6375 West Charleston Boulevard, Suite A-172, Las Vegas, NV 89146, USA
[d] Nevada Tobacco Users' Helpline, University of Nevada School of Medicine, 6375 West Charleston Boulevard, Suite A-172, Las Vegas, NV 89146, USA
[e] UNR Office of Sponsored Projects, 8050 Paradise Road, Suite 125 M/S 0502, Las Vegas, NV 89123, USA
* Corresponding author. School of Nursing, Touro University Nevada, 854 American Pacific Drive, Henderson, NV 89104.
E-mail address: Elizabeth.Fildes@tun.touro.edu

Nurs Clin N Am 47 (2012) 97–107
doi:10.1016/j.cnur.2011.10.009
0029-6465/12/$ – see front matter © 2012 Elsevier Inc. All rights reserved.

prevalence rate of tobacco use, the CDC recommended states to develop a comprehensive plan with the following 4 goals[4]:

- Preventing initiation among youth and young adults
- Promoting quitting among adults and youth
- Eliminating exposure to secondhand smoke
- Identifying and eliminating tobacco-related disparities among population groups

In 2003, the Cessation Subcommittee of the Interagency Committee on Smoking and Health outlined 10 recommendations in the national plan for tobacco cessation. The main goal of these recommendations was to reduce tobacco-related mortality and morbidity in the United States. The first recommendation was to establish a federally funded national tobacco quitline network by 2005.[5]

## Quitlines

Quitlines are telephone-based programs that assist tobacco users to quit. This assistance usually consists of a combination of services including counseling, educational materials on quitting, recorded messages, callbacks from counselors, and smoking cessation medications.[6] In 2009, the North American Quitline Consortium (NAQC), an international professional organization with the mission of promoting evidence-based tobacco cessation quitline services, reported that 515,000 smokers had used quitline services, a 129.7% increase since 2005.[7] At present, quitlines reach between 1% and 2% of all adult smokers.[8]

Starting in September 2012, cigarette package warning labels will display the 1-800-QUIT-NOW telephone number.[9] By putting the 1-800-QUIT-NOW number on cigarette package warning labels, the outreach to smokers with an evidence-based intervention is expected to increase.[10]

## BENEFITS OF QUITLINES

*Treating Tobacco Use and Dependence: 2008 Update. Clinical Practice Guideline* by the US Department of Health and Human Services' Public Health Service identified telephone proactive counseling as an evidence-based treatment that increased the odds of abstinence by approximately 60%.[11] In addition to being evidence based, telephone quitlines have many advantages, including easy accessibility and cost-effectiveness.[6]

## Accessibility

One of the major advantages in using quitlines as a smoking cessation intervention is easy access to help anyone.[6] Being telephone based, quitlines are able to reach tobacco users in remote areas and those with mobility or transportation problems.[12] The semi-anonymous nature of a telephonic setting may also be appealing to tobacco users who are not ready to commit to quitting.[12] Proactive quitlines overcome many of the barriers to cessation programs because they are free and available at the smokers' convenience.[13]

## Cost-Effectiveness

In addition to providing accessible information and assistance to tobacco users, quitlines are also cost-effective.[13] A state quitline is a single centralized operation, with recognizable branding and universal toll-free access.[12] The relatively inexpensive cessation intervention of a centralized quitline is the main reason that many states consider it to be the primary strategy in their statewide cessation program.[12] Some quitlines also provide information and direct referrals to local cessation programs for callers who want to use them.[12]

Quitlines also reduce transportation and childcare costs[13] and eliminate other financial barriers to treatment of those who are uninsured or lack the ability to pay.[13] Delivery of tobacco cessation services by telephone provides services for those populations who may be underserved[4] or disproportionately affected by tobacco use.[4]

### Synergy with Other Tobacco Cessation Interventions

Quitlines are used with other tobacco cessation interventions, including media campaigns and screening programs. Media campaigns that focus on the dangers of smoking and secondhand smoke put pressure on smokers to quit.[12] Quitlines often collaborate with media campaigns to offer assistance to smokers who want to quit.[12] A telephone quitline service is a convenient and easy way for tobacco users to respond to promotional messaging.[6]

The 2008 update to *Treating Tobacco Use and Dependence* recommends that health care providers ask about tobacco use at every visit, advise every tobacco user to quit, and prescribe or recommend US Food and Drug Administration (FDA)–approved medications for every quit attempt in the absence of major medical contraindications.[11] The guideline further suggests that health care providers assist patients to formulate a plan to quit, provide supplementary materials, and schedule a follow-up session to be conducted either in person or by telephone.[11] Offering quitlines as part of a cessation program is an easy and effective way for busy health care professionals to provide a referral service for their patients.[12]

### Access to Multiple Populations

Another component of a comprehensive tobacco control program is to eliminate disparities between various populations regarding tobacco use and access to effective cessation treatment services.[12] With a centralized quitline operation, in which separate language lines can be implemented, it is possible to address disparities.[12] Data from California demonstrate that culturally and linguistically targeted campaigns, tagged with a quitline number, attract smokers of ethnic minority backgrounds as effectively as the general market campaign attracts Caucasian smokers.[6]

## CURRENT QUITLINE OPERATIONS IN THE UNITED STATES

In 2010, the NAQC surveyed 53 US quitlines, 12 Canadian quitlines, 65 funders, and their service providers and determined that 98% of US quitlines provided counseling services 5 days a week for at least 8 hours and 92% provided counseling services on at least 1 weekend day.[14] Furthermore, 92% of US quitlines provided multiple counseling services with a counselor or coach who used proactive calling (ie, the counselor calls the client).[13] Interactive Web-based services varied from offering information about available services, to interactive counseling, to e-mailing.[13] These services were available in multiple languages and often for the hearing impaired.[14] Seventy-five percent of the US quitlines provided free medications, but the type of medications varied.[14] Quitlines were promoted in multiple ways including television (85%), radio (83%), newspaper advertisements (44%), billboards (48%), online advertising (83%), information displays (87%), and health care referral networks (96%).[14]

### Services Available

Most quitlines provide both reactive and proactive calling.[13] Reactive calls provide some form of immediate reactive assistance when a tobacco user first calls, whereas proactive calls are integrative and comprehensive.[12] Proactive calls, initiated by counselors from the quitline, are typically scheduled by agreement with the tobacco user and often entail or result in multiple follow-up sessions.[12] Most quitlines provide multiple proactive counseling sessions, including minimal/brief intervention (33%), single-session counseling (71%), multiple sessions that are initiated by clients (42%), and multiple sessions that are initiated by counselors (92%).[14] Studies have established the effectiveness of proactive interventions; a meta-analysis of 13 studies in 2004 showed a 56% increase in quit rates using proactive interventions compared with self-help.[15]

Quitline services are provided in several languages in the United States, including English (70%), Spanish (56%), Cantonese (1.9%), Mandarin (1.9%), Korean (1.9%), Vietnamese (1.9%), Russian (1.9%), and others (1.9%).[11] Translation services are available from 64% of the US quitlines.[14]

Additional services provided by quitlines include voice mail capability with counselor callbacks (87%), recorded messages for help quitting (69%), mailed information or self-help resources (92%), text messaging to cell phones (4%), and interactive voice responses (2%) and referral to other non-cessation services (62%).[14] Quitlines also offer health care providers multiple methods to refer patients, including fax referral forms, e-mail, and electronic medical records.[14]

To meet the diverse needs of quitline callers, specialized materials for specific populations are distributed based on the caller's needs. These materials include pregnant tobacco users (90%); smokeless tobacco users (90%); various racial/ethnic backgrounds (71%); youth (69%); chronic health conditions (64%); lesbian, gay, bisexual, and transgender (58%); low literacy (12%); young adults (8%); older tobacco users (4%); mental health (4%); multiple addictions (4%); low socioeconomic status (4%); Medicaid (4%); and large print (4%).[14]

### Medication Utilization

Historically, quitlines primarily offered information and/or counseling for tobacco users who wanted to quit.[16] As quitlines grew and budgets increased, quitlines introduced provisions for tobacco cessation medications.[16] In 2008, 36 states offered FDA-approved medications, either free or at discounted rates.[16] At present, 27 states offer nicotine gum, 17 offer nicotine lozenges, and 16 offer both to medically appropriate callers.[16] Four states offer sustained-release bupropion (Zyban) and 2 states offer varenicline (Chantix) free to eligible, medically appropriate callers.[16]

Providing free medication promotes quitline use, motivates tobacco users to quit, increases tobacco abstinence rates, improves caller's satisfaction with the services, and increases the contacts and opportunities for counseling with callers.[16] In considering which medications to offer, quitlines consider the following factors for each client: cost-effectiveness, how easy the medications are to use and/or distribute, drug safety, and side effects.[16]

### Quality Assurance

Public sector quitlines often differ from privately owned quitlines in the scope of their work and in the way services are delivered.[17] Nevertheless, all quitlines share similar responsibilities for providing services, monitoring success, and reporting outcome measures.[17] Furthermore, US quitlines have extensive data collection capabilities, including call volumes, languages used, types of medication distributed, funding sources, media involvement, outreach activities, use of the services, and types of referrals.[14] Client-related data typically collected by all quitlines include the number of clients reached, callers by type of tobacco use, frequency of smoking, gender, age, education levels, race/ethnicity, sexual orientation, insurance types, and client evaluations, including quit rates.[14]

The NAQC has proposed using a quality improvement framework that is currently used in health care settings (the Donabedian framework).[17–19] This framework is useful because it provides information for both the service providers and the funders and incorporates client satisfaction with the services they received, as well as quit rates.[17]

### Funding Sources

State and federal funding for quitline services have increased over the past decade. According to the NAQC, primary quitline funding sources include the CDC, Master Settlement Agreement (MSA) money, and dedicated state tobacco tax funds.[14] Additional funding sources include state Medicaid programs, tobacco settlement funds (non-MSA), charitable foundations, and other nongovernment organizations.[14]

## QUITLINE IN REAL TIME

Although there are many different evidence-based quitline protocols that focus on local resources and needs,[12] it is helpful to have a real-life example of how the quitline intervention is implemented. The Nevada Tobacco Users' Helpline (Helpline) is one example from many US quitlines.

Nevada is far from reaching the 2020 Healthy People goal of reducing the adult smoking rate to 12%. Since 1997, the Helpline has been the state's free tobacco quitline providing comprehensive, statewide nicotine dependence treatment for all forms of tobacco use (smoked and smokeless) and education to all residents aged 18 years and older.

The program is evidence based and adheres to the 2008 update to the *Treating Tobacco Use and Dependence* clinical practice guideline,[11] uses FDA-approved medications, and hires professional counselors for treatment delivery. The Helpline offers an intensive proactive counseling protocol, with many users receiving proactive counseling sessions for a year or more before discharge. The Helpline provides telephone-based nicotine dependence treatment, which includes reactive and proactive counseling sessions. Other services provided by the Helpline include information dissemination regarding nicotine dependence treatment and tobacco use cessation, cessation referrals to in-person programs, and online cessation program resources.

The Helpline data reported here were collected from English-speaking and Spanish-speaking adult residents (18 years and older) of all Nevada counties from July 1, 2010, to June 30, 2011. Institutional review board approval was received from the University of Nevada Reno. From July 1, 2010 to June 30, 2011, the Helpline processed 37,007 calls (**Fig. 1**).

### Service Levels

Callers to the Helpline are offered a variety of services based on the caller's preference and readiness to quit within 30 days.[20] Services are generally classified into 3 levels from least intensive (level I) to most intensive (level III) (**Fig. 2**).

Level I service provides information for individuals inquiring about Helpline services, seeking information on how to quit, or how to help someone else quit, and is considered a minimal intervention. Level I service individuals are typically in the *contemplation* stage of change,[20] considering quitting their tobacco use but not ready to make a quit attempt.

Level II service provides what is considered a brief intervention.[21] A brief intervention for nicotine dependence is a one-time reactive counseling intervention from

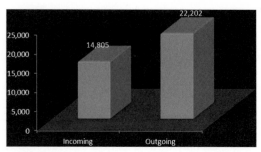

**Fig. 1.** Nevada tobacco users' call volume.

a professional counselor. In the counseling intervention, the counselor addresses the 3 evidence-based strategies of counseling, medication, and support. The caller is mailed a starter kit, which includes an interactive workbook,[22] tailored education materials,[11] and quit referral resources to help the caller make a quit attempt on their own. Individuals who do not wish to speak to a counselor still receive the starter kit.

Level III patients are enrolled in the telephone-based nicotine dependence treatment program and receive multiple proactive and intensive telephone counseling interventions.[23] The term "patient" is used here because the Helpline is part of the Nevada School of Medicine's Department of Psychiatry and offers nicotine dependence treatment. This treatment option is available for 1 year or longer, as needed. Patients receive telephone-based nicotine dependence counseling supported by a psychoeducation program,[24] a medication assistance program (MAP),[25] and a quit kit, which includes a level III booklet, *Living Tobacco Free*.[26] Helpline counselors also provide professional referrals to other allied health professionals, as indicated.

## Treatment

The Helpline treats nicotine dependence using a drug dependency treatment model, viewing tobacco cessation as a process of recovery from nicotine dependence.[27] Professional counselors conceptualize treatment using a solution-focused theoretical approach[28] and motivational interviewing[29] to help move the patient through the stages of change.[30] Solution-focused therapy and motivational interviewing help patients prepare to change by increasing the patient's awareness of the risks of

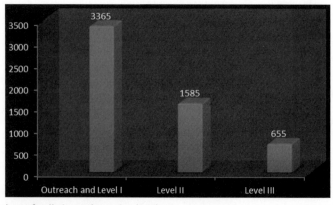

**Fig. 2.** Number of calls in each service level.

tobacco use, the benefits of quitting, their ability to quit tobacco use, and their commitment to the process of nicotine dependence treatment. Counselors also help patients use a wellness paradigm to address how nicotine dependence has affected them physically, emotionally, mentally, and spiritually.

## Holistic Counseling/Total Well-Being

The Helpline's definition of holistic counseling is based on Seaward's description of the wellness paradigm.[31] The Seaward model proposes that total wellness is the balance, integration, and harmony of the physical, emotional, mental, and spiritual aspects of the human condition.[31] The Helpline counselors use the Seward model to implement the following clinical interventions:

- Physical interventions include education and process counseling concerning the risks of tobacco use, the dangers of environmental tobacco smoke, nicotine and the brain, nicotine reduction, 7 delays to tobacco use, setting a quit date, benefits of quitting, withdrawal management, exercise, medication, weight and nutrition management, and trigger management.
- Emotional interventions include education and process counseling concerning emotions, stress management, social support, fear management, anger management, journaling, humor, and joy.
- Mental interventions include education and process counseling concerning cognitive restructuring, assertiveness, communication, self-esteem, affirmations, time management, and relapse management.
- Spiritual interventions include education and process counseling concerning spirituality versus religion, meditation, prayer, nature, exercising the muscles of the soul (ie, expressing gratitude, forgiveness, service, and faith), relationships and acquaintances, purpose, balance, and direction.

## Psychoeducation Program

In addition to treating patients with the wellness paradigm, counselors also use the psychoeducation program, MAP, and the quit kit. The psychoeducation program is provided in a group therapy and/or home study format. The 2 formats are active change agents in treating nicotine dependence and are facilitated by licensed counselors.

Group therapy[24] provides patients with (1) an opportunity to learn new coping techniques and skills from peers; (2) an ability to see personal issues more clearly when expressed by others; and (3) an environment in which tobacco users may feel less defensive and guarded. Group therapy is only available to level III Helpline patients, and there is no limit on the number of therapy sessions attended. During group therapy, patients are assisted in (1) clarifying personal goals, (2) creating and maintaining trust, (3) dealing with fears, and (4) dealing with resistance.

In addition, group therapy has educational objectives in which patients are taught intervention practices on how tobacco/nicotine affects them physically, emotionally, mentally, and spiritually.[31] Supportive and processing group dynamics focus on (1) personal development, (2) enhancement, (3) self-awareness, (4) relapse prevention, and (5) intervention practices that open the doors to growth from a holistic well-being paradigm through sharing how tobacco use and nicotine dependence have affected the patient.[24] The effectiveness of the smoking cessation group therapy has been studied and reported in the literature.[32]

Some patients choose home study over group therapy. Home study is distance education and includes the physical, emotional, mental, and spiritual components of the wellness paradigm. The home study intervention incorporates posttests on each wellness component and they are processed with counselors in a proactive telephone counseling intervention.

## MAP

The MAP provides medication assistance for all types of tobacco use as medically indicated.[11] Current recommendations and patient preferences are discussed with the patient's primary care provider and/or counselor as appropriate. Clients in level III treatment are eligible for FDA-approved medications for tobacco cessation.[25] In 2010 to 2011, 50 of the 122 patients used the MAP within 13 months of initial enrollment.

## Program Evaluation

To collect uniform data, the Helpline uses a minimal data set (MDS) infrastructure that was recommended by the NAQC in 2008.[33] The MDS tool was developed by the Research and Evaluation Workgroup of the NAQC to institute a common framework for communicating about quitline elements and evaluations.[33]

Evaluation of the Helpline's outcomes is currently being conducted by telephone by research assistants. The Helpline secures informed consent from the caller on the first call to the Helpline to collect MDS data and to collect evaluation data at 7 and 13 months. Data are entered into the MDS software and reports are produced quarterly.

At intake, data obtained include demographics, highest level of education, health insurance, employment status, caller's disability, diagnosed conditions (medical, mental, and/or other addictions), tobacco use behaviors, intent to quit, reason for calling, calling for self or on behalf of another, and previous services obtained. Evaluation follow-up data obtained at 7 and 13 months assess caller's satisfaction, current tobacco usage, intent to quit, point prevalence at 7 and 30 days, the last time of smoking, clinical interventions used, medication usage, stage of change, and pregnancy status (**Fig. 3**).

## Quit Rates

One of the most important measures of quitline effectiveness is the quit rate. There are several ways to measure quit rates. The Helpline currently uses a point prevalence abstinence measure, as defined by the NAQC in 2009.[34] The NAQC point prevalence abstinence is the proportion of callers who are abstinent for a designated period of

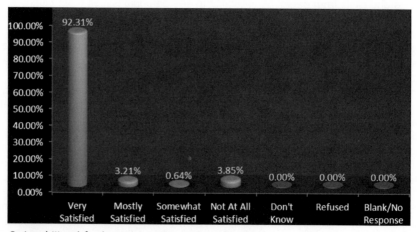

**Fig. 3.** Level III satisfaction rate at 13-month evaluation.

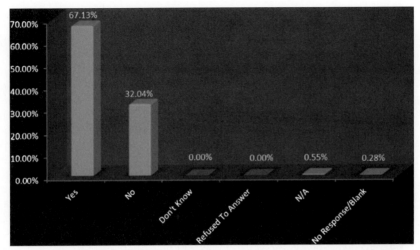

**Fig. 4.** The 30-day point prevalence quit rate for level III was 34.62% at 13 months.

time from immediately before the intervention until the follow-up evaluation. Helpline follow-up evaluations are conducted at 7 and 13 months after the initial day of MDS enrollment, and the Helpline research assistant collects 7-day and 30-day point prevalence abstinence when calling patients (**Fig. 4**).

*Implications for Nurses*

The combination of health professionals referring patients to an accessible, evidence-based, cost-effective cessation resource can produce a substantial reduction in the number of tobacco users in the United States.[35] Quitlines are a great resource for nurses in helping their patients quit tobacco use. The timely and accessible quitline treatment services help tobacco users with significant barriers to traditional face-to-face group counseling, such as transportation difficulties, physical impairment, or work/family responsibilities that would preclude them from attending treatment in a traditional setting.

Only 10% of nurses recommend quitlines to their patients.[36] Initiatives to increase knowledge and working relationships between nurses and quitlines need to be created, implemented, and evaluated.

**ACKNOWLEDGMENTS**

The authors acknowledge Mandy Canales, Project Director; Anastasia Wilson, Evaluation Specialist; Angelica Wilson, Evaluation Specialist; and Corey Coleman, Consultant, Nevada Tobacco Users' Helpline; and all staff members of the Nevada Tobacco Users' Helpline.

**REFERENCES**

1. US Department of Health and Human Services. How tobacco smoke causes disease: the biology and behavioral basis for smoking-attributable disease: a report of the surgeon general. Atlanta (GA): US Department of Health and Human Services, Centers for Disease Control and Prevention, National Center

for Chronic Disease Prevention and Health Promotion, Office on Smoking and Health; 2010. On page 1 of executive summary.

2. Green LW, Ottoson JM. Community and population health. 8th edition. Boston: WCB/McGraw-Hill; 1999.

3. Centers for Disease Control and Prevention. Vital signs: current cigarette smoking among adults aged ≥18 years, United States, 2005–2010. MMWR Morb Mortal Wkly Rep 2011;60(35):1207–12.

4. Centers for Disease Control and Prevention. Best practices for comprehensive tobacco control programs—2007. Atlanta (GA): US Department of Health and Human Services, Centers for Disease Control and Prevention, National Center for Chronic Disease Prevention and Health Promotion, Office on Smoking and Health; 2008.

5. Fiore M, Keller P, Williams L, et al. Preventing 3 million premature deaths and helping 5 million smokers quit: a national action plan for tobacco cessation [serial online]. Am J Public Health 2004;94(2):205–10. Academic Search Premier, Ipswich, MA. Available at: http://ajph.aphapublications.org/cgi/content/full/94/2/205?view=long&pmid=14759928. Accessed August 18, 2011.

6. Lichtenstein E, Shu-Hong Z, Tedeschi GJ. Smoking cessation quitlines. Am Psychol 2010;65(4):252–61. DOI: 10.1037/a001859.

7. North American Quitline Consortium (NAQC). Results from the 2010 NAQC Annual Survey of Quitlines. 2010. Available at: http://www.naquitline.org/?page=survey2010. Accessed July 22, 2011.

8. Cummins SE, Bailey L, Campbell S, et al. Tobacco cessation quitlines in North America: a descriptive study. Tob Control 2007;16(Suppl I):i9–15.

9. Federal Drug Administration (FDA). Cigarette health warnings. Available at: http://www.fda.gov/TobaccoProducts/Labeling/CigaretteWarningLabels/default.htm. Accessed August 18, 2011.

10. North American Quitline Consortium. Health warning labels for tobacco products on June 21, 2011. Available at: http://naquitline.siteym.com/resource/resmgr/Files/NAQC_Talking_Points_FDA_Ruli.pdf. Accessed July 29, 2011.

11. Fiore MC, Jaén CR, Baker TB, et al. Treating tobacco use and dependence: 2008 update. Clinical practice guideline. Rockville (MD): US Department of Health and Human Services. Public Health Service; May 2008.

12. Centers for Disease Control and Prevention. Telephone quitlines: a resource for development, implementation, and evaluation. Final edition. Atlanta (GA): US Department of Health and Human Services, Centers for Disease Control and Prevention, National Center for Chronic Disease Prevention and Health Promotion, Office on Smoking and Health; 2004.

13. Anderson CM, Shu-Hong Z. Tobacco quitlines: looking back and looking ahead. Tob Control 2007;16:i81–6.

14. North American Quitline Consortium. Results from the 2010 NAQC Annual Survey of Quitlines. Webinar presentation July 2011. Available at: http://www.naquitline.org/?page=survey2010. Accessed August 19, 2011.

15. Stead LF, Lancaster T, Perera R. Telephone counseling for smoking cessation (Cochrane Review). Issue 1. In: The Cochrane Library 2004. Chichester (United Kingdom): John Wiley; 2004.

16. Dale L, McAfee T, Tinkelman D, et al. Integration of tobacco cessation medications in state and provincial quitlines: a review of the evidence and the practice with recommendations. Quality improvement initiative. Phoenix (AZ): NAQC; 2009. Available at: http://www.naquitline.org/resource/resmgr/issue_papers/final_layout_version1102.pdf. Accessed August 3, 2011.

17. Michael S. North American Quitline Consortium Quality Improvement Initiative. A framework for improving quality in North America. Phoenix (AZ): NAQC; 2009. Available at: http://www.naquitline.org/resource/resmgr/issue_papers/revisedfinal_framework_paper.pdf. Accessed August 20, 2011.
18. Donabedian A. The definition of quality and approached to its assessment. Ann Arbor (MI): Health Administration Press; 1980.
19. Healthy People 2020. Available at: http://www.healthypeople.gov/2020/topics objectives2020/pdfs/TobaccoUse.pdf. Accessed August 19, 2011.
20. Prochaska JO, DiClemente CC. Stages and processes of self-change of smoking: toward an integrative model of change. J Consult Clin Psychol 1983; 51(3):390–5.
21. Wilson MAT. Nevada Tobacco Users' Helpline guideline for Level II minimal nicotine dependence to adults. CPPW Project. Reno (NV): University of Nevada School of Medicine; 2010.
22. Fildes E, Wilson MAT. Living tobacco free. 2nd edition. Reno (NV): Nevada Tobacco Users' Helpline, University of Nevada School of Medicine; 2009.
23. Wilson MAT. Nevada Tobacco Users Helpline guideline for Level III guideline for nicotine dependence treatment for adults. Reno (NV): University of Nevada School of Medicine; 2010.
24. Corey G. Theory & practice of group counseling. 8th edition. Belmont (CA): Brooks/Cole-Thompson Learning; 2004.
25. Wilson MAT. Nevada Tobacco Users' Helpline guideline for medication assistance program. Reno (NV): University of Nevada School of Medicine; 2010.
26. Fildes E, Skarl S. Your journey to a tobacco-free life. 3rd edition. Las Vegas (NV): Nevada Tobacco Users' Helpline; 2005.
27. American Psychiatric Association. Diagnostic and statistical manual of mental disorders. Text revision. 4th edition. Washington, DC: American Psychiatric Association; 2000.
28. Smock SA, Trepper TS, Wetchler JL, et al. Solution-focused group therapy for Level I substance abusers. J Marital Fam Ther 2008;34(1):107–20. Available at: http://www.solutionfocused.net/f/Solution_Focused_Group_Therapy_for_Level_One_SubstanceAbusers.pdf. Accessed September 22, 2011.
29. Hettema JE, Hendricks PS. Motivational interviewing for smoking cessation: a meta-analytic review. J Consult Clin Psychol 2010;78(6):868–84.
30. Prochaska JO, Norcross JC, DiClemente CC. Changing for good: a revolutionary six-stage program for overcoming bad habits and moving your life forward. New York: William Morrow; 1994.
31. Seaward BL. Managing stress: principles and strategies for health and well being. 5th edition. Sudbury (MA): Jones and Barlett; 2006.
32. Stead LF, Lancaster T. Group behaviour therapy programmes for smoking cessation. Cochrane Database Syst Rev 2005;2:CD001007. DOI: 10.1002/14651858. CD001007.
33. Feltracco A, Saul JE, Davis R, et al. Realizing opportunities: implementation assessment of the minimal data set in North America. Phoenix (AZ): NAQC; 2008.
34. An L, Betzner A, Luxenberg ML, et al. Measuring quit rates. Quality improvement initiative. Phoenix (AZ): NAQC; 2009. Available at: http://www.naquitline.org/resource/resmgr/docs/naqc_issuepaper_measuringqui.pdf. Accessed August 16, 2011.
35. Sarna L, Bialous SA, Rice VH, et al. Promoting tobacco dependence treatment in nursing education. Drug Alcohol Rev 2009;28(5):507–16.
36. Sarna L, Bialous SA, Wells M, et al. Frequency of nurses' smoking cessation interventions: report from a national survey. J Clin Nurs 2009;18(14):2066–77.

# The Three Ts of Adopting Tobacco-free Policies on College Campuses

Ellen J. Hahn, PhD, RN[a],*, Amanda Fallin, PhD, RN[b],
Audrey Darville, APRN, CTTS[a],[c], Sarah E. Kercsmar, PhD[a],[d],
Melissa McCann[a], Rachael A. Record, MA[a],[d]

**KEYWORDS**

• Tobacco • Policy • Smoking cessation • Smoke-free

Exposure to secondhand smoke (SHS) is a known serious cause of preventable disease and premature death, including lung cancer, coronary heart disease and myocardial infarction,[1] and respiratory complications.[2,3] Within 5 minutes of exposure, SHS makes it harder for the heart to pump blood. In about 25 minutes, fat and blood clots build up in the arteries, increasing the chance of heart attack and stroke. After only 2 hours of exposure to SHS, the heart rate speeds up and leads to abnormal heart rhythms (which can be fatal).[4] Even outdoor exposure to SHS presents health risks.[5,6]

---

Funding: Funding was provided by the University of Kentucky President's Office through the Office of the Executive Vice President for Finance and Administration. This publication was supported by grant number UL1RR033173 from the National Center for Research Resources (NCRR), funded by the Office of the Director, National Institutes of Health (NIH) and supported by the NIH Roadmap for Medical Research (E. Hahn, Co-Investigator). The content is solely the responsibility of the authors and does not necessarily represent the official views of NCRR and NIH.

Disclosures: Ellen J. Hahn is the Co-Chair of the University of Kentucky Tobacco-free Task Force and Co-investigator, UK Center for Clinical and Translational Science (UL1RR033173); Audrey Darville is a certified tobacco treatment specialist and she provides tobacco treatment services for UKHealthCare. The other authors have no conflicts of interest, financial or otherwise, to disclose.

[a] Kentucky Center for Smoke-free Policy, Tobacco Policy Research Program, University of Kentucky College of Nursing, 751 Rose Street, Lexington, KY 40536-0232, USA
[b] Center for Tobacco Control Research and Education, University of California San Francisco, 530 Parnassus Avenue, San Francisco, CA 94143, USA
[c] UKHealthCare, 800 Rose Street, Lexington, KY 40536, USA
[d] Kentucky Center for Smoke-free Policy, University of Kentucky College of Communications and Information Studies, Little Library 310 M, Lexington, KY 40536, USA
* Corresponding author.
*E-mail address:* ejhahn00@email.uky.edu

doi:10.1016/j.cnur.2011.11.002
0029-6465/12/$ – see front matter
**nursing.theclinics.com**

Nationwide, colleges, universities, and health care campuses recognize the health threat from SHS and there is a trend toward implementing tobacco-free or smoke-free campus policies.[7] As of October 7, 2011, there were at least 586 US colleges or universities with 100% smoke-free or tobacco-free campus policies with no exemptions.[8] Although there has been a recent wave of tobacco-free campuses in the United States, policy restrictiveness and implementation vary, and compliance remains a challenge. Streets and sidewalks not owned or controlled by the college or university create special challenges. This case study describes the 3 Ts strategy to implementing and evaluating the University of Kentucky's (UK's) tobacco-free campus policy and evaluates the outcomes and costs.

## HISTORY/CONTEXT OF POLICY

UK, located in Lexington, joined the list of higher-education institutions with a tobacco-free campus policy in November 2009.[8] As the state's land grant university, UK is located in a state that is a national leader in tobacco production.[9] Given the historically protobacco climate,[10] the adoption and implementation of the policy did not come quickly; nor was there immediate adherence. However, there was administrative support for the policy from the beginning. The campus went tobacco-free in stages. First, the academic medical center campus, adjacent to the main campus, went tobacco-free in November 2008, exactly 1 year before the entire campus implemented its comprehensive tobacco-free policy. Great American SmokeOut[11] was selected as the implementation date for both the medical center and the entire campus policy.

In both cases, UK spent about 9 to 12 months in the preparation phase to promote buy-in from key stakeholders, including tobacco users, and to develop a strong implementation plan using a 3-pronged 3-Ts approach: tell, treat, and train. Integrated, regular, consistent communications (tell) were critical to creating an environment in which compliance was expected. Given that policy change increases demand for tobacco treatment,[12–15] providing evidence-based tobacco treatment (treat) was an important hallmark of the policy strategy. Effective policy implementation relied on well-trained administrators, faculty, and student leaders (train) to remind violators of the policy and report if necessary. The 3 Ts approach is designed to institute a culture of policy compliance.

The Tobacco-free Campus Task Force (TCTF), representing 28 sectors of the university community, including faculty, staff, and students, was appointed by the University President about 11 months before implementation of the campus-wide policy. The group initially met semiweekly and they formed 5 committees that met consistently during the 10-month planning period. About 200 people were involved in the planning and they were invited to a kick-off event hosted by the President and TCTF. The communication plan involved integrating the tobacco-free policy message into all new (and prospective) student, faculty, and staff orientation activities, alumni and parents' materials, athletic ticket materials and events, and various campus publications, as well as communicating via Web sites, email broadcasts, brochures, table tents in dining areas, parking tickets, and campus print, television, and radio media.

Existing vendors and contractors were notified and all contracts included policy language and expectations. Tobacco treatment services for employees and students were enhanced and available 30 to 60 days before the policy implementation date. Little research was available to assist the TCTF and the planning committees with effective policy development and enforcement strategies. Despite the recent wave of tobacco-free colleges,[7] there is little research on campus policy strategies, effectiveness, and enforcement procedures.

## THE 3 Ts STRATEGY: TELL

The first component of the 3-pronged approach is tell. For successful policy implementation, adequate and timely notification about the policy provisions is crucial. Communication about the policy was a top priority before policy implementation. Throughout campus, signs were placed in strategic outdoor locations and in places where pedestrians and vehicles entered campus. The signs were designed with a positive message including the rationale for the policy: "Welcome to our Tobacco Free Campus: A Healthy Place to Live, Work and Learn." Signage was periodically evaluated and replaced because of damage or vandalism.

Shortly before the policy went into effect, an email from the University President about the policy was sent to students and employees. The message described the need to create a healthy campus environment and information about how to obtain tobacco treatment services. Employees were invited to a 2-day resource fair hosted by the College of Nursing's Tobacco Policy Research Program before the policy went into effect. Employees were provided with information about BeHIP, a phone-based coaching program for those who wished to quit using tobacco products, individual counseling sessions with the university's tobacco treatment specialist, and visits to the office of UK Work + Life Connections, which provided employees with tobacco education, assessments, and referrals free of charge. Students were provided with information on tobacco cessation options and prescriptions through University Health Services (UHS) and counseling programs through the university's Counseling and Testing Center. Two brochures were distributed at key campus locations: one brochure contained information about the policy and the boundaries, and the other emphasized various tobacco treatment resource options (see http://www.uky.edu/Tobaccofree).

Before and after the policy went into effect, the cochairs of the TCTF conducted road shows with employee and student groups (eg, library employee group, staff and faculty senates, arts and sciences student ambassadors). A 15-minute slide presentation introduced the policy (including specific boundaries), resources available for students and employees who wished to quit using tobacco, consequences for violating the policy, and answered questions and concerns. In 2011 (nearly 2 years after policy implementation), information about the tobacco-free policy and tobacco treatment services was added to the course content for UK 101, a class for incoming freshman that acquaints the student with campus during their first semester.

Clear communication is particularly important when discussing policy boundaries. For example, the tobacco-free policy does not cover city-owned or state-owned sidewalks or streets, creating confusion when smokers congregate in areas that may seem to be on campus. The TCTF published the following statement related to these areas: "For those sidewalks adjacent to streets not controlled by the university, we ask that you respect the pedestrians and our efforts to provide a healthier environment by refraining from tobacco use on those sidewalks." This statement was integrated into the maps of policy boundaries.

In the 2 years after implementation, it has been important to continue and repeat tell strategies. Anniversary events raised awareness about the policy. UHS distributed cold turkey sandwiches ("You need more than cold turkey to quit") and s'mores ("Ask us s'more about quitting") in high-traffic campus areas. Policy reminder cards with a positive message including a coupon for a free fountain drink (eg, iced tea, lemonade, soft drinks) were distributed in high-traffic areas and during busy times (ie, class change times).[16] Media stories in the student newspaper and on radio attracted interest from students completing individual and group class projects.

## THE 3 Ts STRATEGY: TREAT

Providing evidence-based tobacco treatment services[17] is the second element of the 3 Ts strategy. Cessation strategies are most effective when there is a combination of medication, counseling, smoke-free policy, cigarette tax increases, and media education. Tailored approaches to medication and counseling are most effective in helping people quit tobacco use.[17] UK followed the 2008 Update of the Clinical Practice Guidelines for Treating Tobacco Use and Dependence as a framework[17] for enhancing and developing tobacco treatment programs for students and employees before and during implementation of the tobacco-free campus policy. Based on these guidelines, a variety of cessation group and individual counseling options are offered to students, employees, and sponsored dependents covered on the university health plan. Cessation medications (ie, combination nicotine replacement therapy [NRT], including patches plus gum or lozenges) are made available for free for persons participating in one of the cessation programs.

The existing employee health and wellness program, a structured, telephone-based cessation counseling program including NRT products and a personal health coach, was expanded because of the anticipated and actual increase in program participation after the tobacco-free campus policy went into effect. Employees also have access to individualized counseling at UKHealthCare by a nurse practitioner who is also a certified tobacco treatment specialist. Individual counseling is available in person and via phone, email, or online support. Sessions provide motivational counseling, development of tailored treatment approaches, and the use of medications approved by the US Food and Drug Administration.[17] Group sessions are also available in partnership with the local health department's ongoing group tobacco cessation classes. To maximize access to treatment, counseling services are provided at varying times of the day and evening. Students have access to tobacco use treatment through UHS and the student counseling center. In these settings, a nurse practitioner, health education specialist, and psychologist provide individualized cessation counseling and treatment. To receive a 2-week coupon for free NRT patches, gum, or lozenges, students and employees are required to participate in some form of a structured cessation program.

The TCTF delegated the responsibility for enhancing existing services and creating a coordinated tobacco treatment program to the Tobacco Dependence Treatment Committee, including members of student health, counseling services, health and wellness, employee benefits, health care, and faculty, students, and the tobacco control specialist from the local health department. Three of the committee members were certified tobacco treatment specialists.

A campus-wide online survey to assess prevalence of tobacco use and interest in quitting resources among students and employees was conducted 6 months before policy implementation. Given that nearly one-third expressed interest in quitting, there was a documented need to enhance tobacco cessation support. Given the number of tobacco users on campus and in an effort to promote compliance, low-cost NRT products were available for purchase at multiple convenient campus locations. The message to users who may not be ready to quit was that they could be comfortable while on campus by using nicotine gum or patches.

A variety of media were used to promote the tobacco treatment services. Committee members were interviewed by the student newspaper and radio station. Print materials and posters were developed and distributed during special campus events, including a campus house calls event, in which information on campus services was provided to students individually in their dormitories. This information included messages such as "Picture Yourself Tobacco Free," and "iThink, iQuit, iConquer" themed materials developed by the UHS Health Education Specialist. The tobacco-free Web site (http://www.uky.edu/Tobaccofree) provided a comprehensive listing of treatment resources for students, employees, and community members. Bulletins, emails and newsletters included information about the tobacco treatment services and they were distributed through Employee Benefits, Health and Wellness, and UKHealthCare programs.

## THE 3 Ts STRATEGY: TRAIN

The third prong of the 3 Ts strategy to tobacco-free policy development is to train supervisors, faculty, administrators, and student leaders on the policy and how to approach violators. The goal of the train component is to create a culture of policy compliance so that enforcing the tobacco-free rules is everyone's job. Approaching violators can be intimidating, so providing tools is one way to increase compliance with the policy, in addition to tell and treat approaches.

Before the policy went into effect, training was provided to promote compliance with the policy. A slide presentation included proper scripting to use when approaching violators of the tobacco-free policy. Given that compliance is everyone's business, employees or students were asked to politely but firmly remind the violator about the policy and potential consequences, and ask them to extinguish or dispose of the tobacco product using the scripted messages.

All members of campus were asked to: (1) introduce yourself and your role on campus; (2) remind the violator about the tobacco-free policy; (3) politely but firmly ask them to extinguish and dispose of the tobacco product; and (4) inform them of low-cost NRT available at multiple convenient campus locations to minimize cravings and promote comfort (**Table 1**). As part of the training protocol, employees and students are provided with a map of the campus boundaries and information on tobacco treatment services.

For those who refuse to comply with the policy, students are reported to the Dean of Students for violating the Student Code of Conduct (Part 1, Article 2, Prohibited Conduct: "Violation of other published University regulations or policies"). Possible sanctions for the student violator included a disciplinary warning, reprimand or probation, social suspension, and disciplinary suspension or expulsion depending on the magnitude of the violation (Part 1, Article 2, Sanctions). Faculty and staff who violate

| Table 1 | | |
| --- | --- | --- |
| **Example of scripting used with violators of the tobacco-free policy** | | |
| **Type** | **Script Example** | |
| Scenario I: | "Hello, my name is _____, and I am an (employee /student) here at UK. Are you aware that our campus is tobacco-free? This means I'm going to have to ask you to put your cigarette out and dispose of it in the trash can. Thank you for respecting our policy. There are locations on campus that sell nicotine replacement for a discounted price so you can be comfortable on campus." | |

the policy are reported to their manager or academic dean. Employee violations are treated as any other infraction of campus policy and are dealt with through corrective action. Repeat offenders are subject to possible termination of employment.

Eighteen months after the policy was implemented, the TCTF launched an ambassador program to more deliberately create an environment of compliance. The Tobacco-free Take Action! Ambassador program is comprised of employees and students who are proactive in increasing compliance with the tobacco-free policy. Specific hot spots where policy violators congregate are identified through cigarette butt clean-up efforts and complaints to the TCTF, and they are deliberately targeted for proactive hot spot interventions.

Ambassadors complete training on how to use a firm, yet compassionate approach to violators by using scripted messages. They also learn how to report violators who continue to violate after reminded. Ambassadors are required to show competence in scripting through role playing before they are assigned to hot spots. Ambassadors are assigned to hot spots in teams of 2 and they target a spot for 20 minutes during class change or at other high-traffic times. They approach violators and complete a site-specific checklist assessing number of male and female violators observed, number of violators approached, how the violator responded (eg, immediately extinguished tobacco product, ignored ambassador), and action taken by the ambassador (ie, reported to Dean of Students or supervisor). If a violator refuses to comply with the policy when reminded, the ambassador asks for identification and reports them according to approved compliance procedures (see http://www.uky.edu/Tobaccofree).

## EVALUATION OF OUTCOMES AND COSTS

Quit attempts among students and employees have increased since the campus-wide tobacco-free policy took effect. Based on use of the free NRT benefit, a total of 335 persons received tobacco dependence treatment during the 2-year period after the policy took effect, compared with only 33 in the year preceding the campus-wide policy (**Table 2**). On average, about 3 tobacco users sought cessation services per month before the campus-wide policy, compared to 11 per month after policy implementation, reflecting a 4-fold increase in demand for tobacco treatment services. Of the 263 enrolled in tobacco treatment services, 48% were employees, 46% were students, and 6% were spouses/sponsored dependents and retirees. Before the

| Table 2 | | | | | | |
|---------|--|--|--|--|--|--|
| Cessation Program Participation and Nicotine Replacement (NRT) Use Over Time | | | | | | |
| | 1 Year Before Policy 11/08–10/09 | November 09–March 2010 | April–September 2010 | October 10–March 2011 | April–September 2011 | Total Post-Policy |
| Enrolled in Program | 33 | 116 | 86 | 87 | 105 | 263 |
| NRT Coupons | 124 | 272 | 198 | 221 | 284 | 975 |
| Cost of NRT (US$) | $5902.37 | $5096.43 | $3979.46 | $3595.11 | $4046.20 | $16,717.20 |

*Note.* The total post-policy number enrolled reflects unique patients. Students, employees, and sponsored dependents are eligible to receive free NRT for 12 weeks (distributed in 2-week coupons).

| Table 3 Tobacco Use Patterns of Cessation Program Survey Respondents (*N* = 36) | | | | | | | |
|---|---|---|---|---|---|---|---|
| | Current Tobacco User/ Quit < 7 days | | Quit 8–30 days | | Quit > 30 days | | Total Responses |
| | n | (%) | n | (%) | n | (%) | N |
| Students | 7 | (38.9) | 0 | (0.0) | 4 | (30.8) | 11 |
| Employees | 11 | (61.1) | 5 | (100.0) | 9 | (69.2) | 25 |
| Total | 18 | (50.0) | 5 | (13.9) | 13 | (36.1) | 36 |

policy, the average number of NRT coupons redeemed per month was 10, compared to 41 per month after the policy was implemented, representing a 4-fold increase in coupons redeemed. The cost associated with NRT coupons increased from $491.86 per month before the policy to $696.55 per month after the policy took effect, reflecting only a 1.4-fold increase in cost. These cost savings were because of a lower cost per NRT coupon after the policy negotiated by UK Pharmacy, from $47.60 per coupon before the policy to $17.15 per coupon on average after the policy.

A follow-up survey was conducted via email with tobacco treatment program participants 16 months after the tobacco-free campus policy was implemented to assess tobacco use, cessation methods used, and quit status. A total of 207 surveys were emailed to participating students, faculty, and staff, and 36 were returned after 2 reminder emails (17% participation rate). Of the 36 surveys, 25 were employees and 11 were students; 61% were females. The low response rate limits the generalizability of the analysis, but there are some interesting trends.

Of the 36 participants, 18 (50%) were current tobacco users. Using an intent-to-treat analysis in which nonrespondents are considered tobacco users, the quit rate for the sample of 207 program participants was 8.7%. Thirty respondents (83%) reported smoking cigarettes in the past year, with an average of 14 cigarettes smoked per day (range = 1 to 35 daily). Other tobacco products used included smokeless (8%), cigars (6%), and hookah (6%). Both students and employees reported relatively high levels of confidence in quitting, and these groups did not differ in confidence to quit; mean values were 7.3 ± 2.8 and 7.5 ± 2.7, respectively (0 = not at all to 10 = extremely confident). Both groups reported even greater confidence that they could remain tobacco free while on campus (students 8.4 ± 3.2; employees 8.3 ± 2.8).

Overall, nearly three-fourths of those who had quit using tobacco reported being abstinent for more than 30 days (**Table 3**). Of those who were unable to quit, nearly half of them reported that they reduced their tobacco use by 50% or more. Regardless of whether or not they quit, nearly all (92%) used NRT; only 8% used Chantix (2 quit and 1 did not). Given the low overall response rate and small sample size, it is difficult to determine cessation outcomes. Considering these limitations, the evaluation data on cessation and cigarette reduction rates should be interpreted with caution.

Although observed and reported smoking has declined since the policy took effect, evidence of cigarette butts remains.[18] The recent launch of the Tobacco-free Take Action! Ambassador program aims to improve compliance. Early observations show promise in the effectiveness of the program, but evaluation data are not yet available.

## SUMMARY

This case study described the 3 Ts (tell-treat-train) strategy, designed to institute a culture of policy compliance, and evaluated its impact on outcomes and costs. The 3 Ts strategy involves regular, consistent communications, access to tobacco treatment medications and counseling, and ongoing training of supervisors and student leaders. Sustained, clear communications using multiple channels targeting students, employees, visitors, and vendors is essential to successful policy implementation (tell). Providing access to free or low-cost evidence-based tobacco treatment services by qualified personnel is important for meeting the demand for tobacco cessation (treat). For users who were not ready to quit, low-cost NRT products were available for purchase at multiple convenient campus locations to promote symptom management while on campus. Creating a climate of policy compliance is also achieved by initial as well as ongoing training of supervisors and student leaders about the policy and how best to approach violators using a firm, yet compassionate approach (train). Demand for tobacco treatment services increased, from an average of 3 enrolled in cessation programs per month before the campus-wide policy to 11 per month after the policy took effect, representing a 4-fold increase in quit attempts. During this period, 975 free nicotine replacement coupons (2-week supply) were redeemed, a 4-fold increase in treatment use, for a total postpolicy cost of $16,717. Although the intent-to-treat estimated quit rate was only 8.7%, both students and employees reported high levels of confidence that they could remain tobacco free while on campus. NRT was the medication of choice, likely because the university covered the full cost of the medication for 12 weeks. Of treatment participants sampled ($N = 36$) and unable to quit, nearly half of them reported they had reduced their tobacco use by 50% or more. Administrative support, access to tobacco treatment, campus buy-in, sustained communications, and careful implementation planning are critical to instituting a tobacco-free university policy.

## ACKNOWLEDGMENTS

We acknowledge Frank Butler, Executive Vice President for Finance and Administration, for consistent and strong support of the policy and for his service as administration liaison; Lucy B. Wells RPh, UK Prescription Benefits and member UK Tobacco Task Force, for supplying the nicotine replacement use data; and Anthany Beatty, VP for Campus Services, Co-Chair, Tobacco Task Force, for his leadership in planning and implementing the tobacco-free policy.

## REFERENCES

1. Institute of Medicine. Secondhand smoke exposure and cardiovascular effects: making sense of the evidence. Washington, DC: The National Academies Press; 2010.
2. US Department of Health and Human Services. How tobacco smoke causes disease: the biology and behavioral basis for smoking-attributable disease: a report of the surgeon general. Atlanta (GA): US Department of Health and Human Services, Centers for Disease Control and Prevention, National Center for Chronic Disease Prevention and Health Promotion, Office on Smoking and Health; 2010.
3. US Department of Health and Human Services. The health consequences of involuntary exposure to tobacco smoke: a report of the surgeon general. Atlanta (GA): Department of Health and Human Services, Public Health Service, Centers for Disease Control and Prevention, National Center for Chronic Disease and Prevention and Promotion, Office of Smoking and Health; 2006.
4. Otsuka R, Watanabe H, Hirata K, et al. Acute effects of passive smoking on the coronary circulation in healthy young adults. JAMA 2001;286(4):436–41.

5. Hall JC, Bernert JT, Hall DB, et al. Assessment of exposure to secondhand smoke at outdoor bars and family restaurants in Athens, Georgia, using salivary cotinine. J Occup Environ Hyg 2009;6(11):698–704.
6. Klepeis NE, Ott WR, Switzer P. Real-time measurement of outdoor tobacco smoke particles. J Air Waste Manag Assoc 2007;57(5):522–34.
7. Lee JGL, Goldstein AO, Kramer KD, et al. Statewide diffusion of 100% tobacco-free college and university policies. Tob Control 2010;19(4):311.
8. Americans for Nonsmokers' Rights. U.S. Colleges and universities with smokefree air policies. 2011. Available at: http://no-smoke.org/pdf/smokefreecollegesuniversities. pdf. Accessed October 23, 2011.
9. US Department of Agriculture. Data and statistics, crops and plants, tobacco (all classes). 2010. Available at: http://www.nass.usda.gov/QuickStats. Accessed July 1, 2011.
10. Chaloupka F, Hahn E, Emery S. Policy levers for the control of tobacco consumption. Kentucky Law J 2002;90(4):1009–42.
11. Centers for Disease Control and Prevention. Great American Smokeout–November 16, 2000. MMWR 2000;49(3):977.
12. Moskowitz JM, Lin Z, Hudes ES. The impact of workplace smoking ordinances in California on smoking cessation. Am J Public Health 2000;90(5):757–61.
13. Tauras JA. Public policy and smoking cessation among young adults in the United States. Health Policy 2004;68(3):321–32.
14. Ripley-Moffitt C, Viera AJ, Goldstein AO, et al. Influence of a tobacco-free hospital campus policy on smoking status of hospital employees. Am J Health Promot 2010;25(1):e25–8.
15. Metzger KB, Mostashari F, Kerker BD. Use of pharmacy data to evaluate smoking regulations' impact on sales of nicotine replacement therapies in New York City. Am J Public Health 2005;95(6):1050–5.
16. Fallin A, Johnson AO, Riker CA, et al. An intervention to increase compliance with a tobacco-free university policy. Lexington (KY): University of Kentucky College of Nursing; 2011.
17. Fiore M, Jaén C, Baker T, et al. Treating tobacco use and dependence: 2008 update. Rockville (MD): US Department of Health and Human Services, Public Health Service; 2008.
18. Fallin A, Murrey M, Johnson AO, et al. Measuring compliance with tobacco-free campus policy. Lexington (KY): University of Kentucky College of Nursing; 2011.

# Preventing Adolescent Tobacco Use and Assisting Young People to Quit: Population-, Community-, and Individually Focused Evidence-Based Interventions

Diana P. Hackbarth, RN, PhD[a,b,c],*

KEYWORDS

- Adolescent smoking • Tobacco use prevention
- Smoking cessation • Tobacco control • Tobacco marketing

The tobacco epidemic kills almost 6 million people worldwide each year. Of these, approximately 5 million are tobacco users and the remainder die from exposure to secondhand smoke.[1] In the United States, cigarette smoking remains the leading cause of preventable morbidity and mortality, responsible for an estimated 443,000 premature deaths and $193 billion in direct health care expenditures and productivity losses each year.[2] Most people who become regular tobacco users begin using tobacco products at or before adolescence. The number of persons aged 12 or older who smoked cigarettes for the first time within the past 12 months was 2.4 million in 2008 but significantly higher than the estimate for 2002 (1.9 million). The 2008 estimate averages out to approximately 6600 new cigarette smokers every day. Most new cigarette smokers in 2008 were under age 18 when they first smoked cigarettes (58.8 percent).[3] The vast majority of persons who begin smoking during adolescence are addicted to nicotine by age 20.[4]

Conflicts of interest: none.
[a] Infection Prevention MSN & DNP, Niehoff School of Nursing, Loyola University Chicago, 2160 South First Avenue, Maywood, IL 60153, USA
[b] School-based Health Center at Proviso East High School, Maywood, IL, USA
[c] Illinois Coalition Against Tobacco, Chicago, IL, USA
* Infection Prevention MSN & DNP, Niehoff School of Nursing, Loyola University Chicago, 2160 South First Avenue, Maywood, IL 60153.
E-mail address: dhackba@luc.edu

Nurs Clin N Am 47 (2012) 119–140
doi:10.1016/j.cnur.2011.10.004
0029-6465/12/$ – see front matter © 2012 Elsevier Inc. All rights reserved.

nursing.theclinics.com

Tobacco use by adolescents is a unique public health problem. Tobacco is the only consumer product that, when used as directed, sickens and kills its users. In addition, new consumers must be recruited by the tobacco industry and become addicted in order for there to be a continuing market. According to US District Judge Gladys Kessler, in her opinion in US v Philip Morris,[5] "From the 1950s to the present, different defendants, at different times and using different methods, have intentionally marketed to young people under the age of twenty-one to recruit 'replacement smokers' to ensure the economic future of the tobacco industry." Therefore, to understand evidence-based interventions to prevent adolescent tobacco use or to help young smokers quit, the role of the multibillion dollar, multinational tobacco industry in continuing to promote tobacco products and in undermining global public health efforts to control tobacco use must be appreciated.

Organized efforts to reduce the burden of tobacco-related disease and youth access to tobacco exist globally, nationally, and at the state and local levels. The Framework Convention on Tobacco Control (FCTC)[6] is the first global public health treaty negotiated by the World Health Organization (WHO) and currently has been ratified by 174 countries. It outlines global strategies to protect young people from becoming tobacco users and/or from being exposed to secondhand smoke. **Box 1** contains the objectives and core demand and supply reduction provisions of the FCTC. More information can be found at http://www.who.int/fctc/en.

In the United States, there are many laws and regulations at the federal, state, and local levels enacted to control tobacco use. In November 2010, the US Department of Health and Human Services (DHHS) released a report entitled, "Ending the Tobacco Epidemic: A Tobacco Control Strategic Action Plan," with a goal to create

---

**Box 1**
**FCTC objectives and core demand and supply reduction provisions**

The objective of this Convention and its protocols is to protect present and future generations from the devastating health, social, environmental, and economic consequences of tobacco consumption and exposure to tobacco smoke by providing a framework for tobacco control measures to be implemented by the parties at the national, regional, and international levels to reduce continually and substantially the prevalence of tobacco use and exposure to tobacco smoke.

The core demand reduction provisions in the WHO FCTC are contained in articles 6 to 14:

- Price and tax measures to reduce the demand for tobacco

- Nonprice measures to reduce the demand for tobacco, namely

  o Protection from exposure to tobacco smoke

  o Regulation of the contents of tobacco products

  o Regulation of tobacco product disclosures

  o Packaging and labeling of tobacco products

  o Education, communication, training, and public awareness

  o Tobacco advertising, promotion, and sponsorship

  o Demand reduction measures concerning tobacco dependence and cessation

The core supply reduction provisions in the WHO FCTC are contained in articles 15 to 17:

- Illicit trade in tobacco products

- Sales to and by minors

- Provision of support for economically viable alternative activities

a society free of tobacco-related death and disease.[7] This plan emphasizes tobacco control measures at the population, community, and individual levels. Its objectives and strategies complement the WHO's global initiative outlined in the FCTC. Healthy People 2020 is the Centers for Disease Control and Prevention's blueprint for enhancing the health status of all people in the United States. This document identifies reducing tobacco use as a priority to meet the national goal of a society in which all people live long, healthy lives.[8] Healthy People 2020 provides a framework for understanding tobacco use prevention among adolescents and evidence-based interventions to encourage cessation. The Healthy People 2020 model assumes that there are many determinants that contribute to health and disease in populations. These include biology and genetics, individual behavior, social environment, physical environment, and access to health services. Specific Healthy People 2020 objectives focusing on tobacco and youth are summarized in **Box 2**.[8]

Based on the FCTC and strategies outlined in the "Ending the Tobacco Epidemic" plan and the Healthy People 2020 model of health determinants, effective strategies to reduce adolescent tobacco use must go beyond individually focused interventions and/or group health education or cessation programs. **Box 3** lists the Healthy People 2020 framework to end the tobacco use epidemic. Some interventions do address adolescent tobacco use at the biologic/genetic and individual levels and include a role for health care providers in delivering evidence-based programs. The framework emphasizes society-wide interventions, however, to change the social and physical environments to prevent young people from starting to smoke and make it easier for adolescents and adults to quit.

## SCOPE OF ADOLESCENT TOBACCO USE IN THE UNITED STATES

The prevalence of cigarette smoking among youth and adult smokers has declined, but that decline has stalled during the past 5 years among adults.[9] This is illustrated in **Fig. 1**.

---

**Box 2**
**Healthy People 2020 objectives for reducing tobacco exposure and use by adolescents**

TU-2 Reduce tobacco use by adolescents.

TU-3 Reduce the initiation of tobacco use among children, adolescents, and young adults.

TU-7 Increase smoking cessation attempts by adolescent smokers. Increase smoking cessation attempts by adolescent smokers.

TU-11 Reduce the proportion of nonsmokers exposed to secondhand smoke.

TU-14 Increase the proportion of smoke-free homes. Increase the proportion of smoke-free homes.

TU-15 Increase tobacco-free environments in schools, including all school facilities, property, vehicles, and school events.

TU-16 Eliminate state laws that preempt stronger local tobacco control laws, including laws that limit youth access to tobacco products.

TU-18 Reduce the proportion of adolescents and young adults, grades 6 through 12, who are exposed to tobacco advertising and promotion.

TU-19 Reduce the illegal sales rate to minors through enforcement of laws prohibiting the sale of tobacco products to minors.

*Abbreviation:* TU, tobacco use.

| Box 3 |
| --- |
| **Healthy People 2020 framework for ending tobacco use epidemic** |
| • Fully funding tobacco control programs |
| • Increasing the price of tobacco products |
| • Enacting comprehensive smoke-free policies |
| • Controlling access to tobacco products |
| • Reducing tobacco advertising and promotion |
| • Implementing antitobacco media campaigns |
| • Encouraging and assisting tobacco users to quit |

In the United States, periodic surveys are conducted to estimate the prevalence of tobacco use among youth.[10,11] These surveys monitor priority health risk behaviors among youth and adults in the United States. The YRBS is conducted every 2 years and provides data representative of 9th-grade through 12th-grade students in public and private schools throughout the United States. In 2009, 46.3% of adolescents had tried smoking, 19.5% had smoked a cigarette within the last 30 days, and 7.3% smoked on 20 or more days in the month previous to the survey. In addition, 8.9% had used chewing tobacco, snuff, or dip on at least 1 day and 14% smoked cigars or little cigars on at least 1 day before the survey. Tobacco use varied between gender groups and racial/ethnic groups. For example, among black students, 9.5% smoked at least 1 cigarette a day in the 30 days before the survey compared with 18% of Hispanic students. In contrast, white students reported the highest rate of smoking at least one cigarette in the 30-day period, 22.5%. Differences by gender were

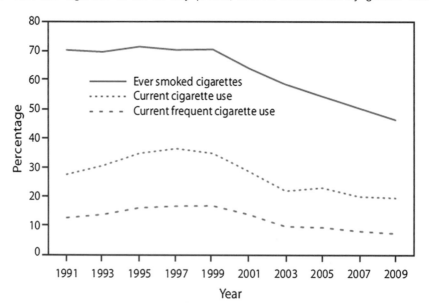

**Fig. 1.** Percentage of high school students who had ever smoked cigarettes, were current cigarette users, and were current frequent cigarette users—Youth Risk Behavior Survey, United States, 1991–2009. (*From* Centers for Disease Control and Prevention. Cigarette use among high school students—United States, 1991–2009. MMWR Morb Mortal Wkly Rep 2010;59(27):797–801.)

reported, with 6.4% of girls reporting smoking on 20 or more days compared with 8% of boys. Not surprisingly, girls were less likely to use chewing tobacco than boys with rates of 2.2% and 15%, respectively. Regional differences in tobacco use among youth also exist, with only 24% of adolescents in Utah reporting ever having tried cigarette smoking compared with 53% in South Carolina. The surveys also indicated that 22.2% of participants nationally reported using marijuana 1 or more times in the 30 days before the survey, a percentage comparable to tobacco use.[10] The National Survey on Drug Use and Health also captures data on youth smoking and may include young people not currently in school. "Current smoker" in this survey included persons who had smoked at least 1 cigarette in the 30 days before the 2006–2008 National Survey on Drug Use and Health. Prevalence of smoking among youths age 12 to 17 was estimated to be 11.8% among white non-Hispanics, 5.9% among black non-Hispanics, 7.4% among Hispanics, and 4.1% among Asian youth. The ethnic group with the highest smoking prevalence among youth was American Indians/Alaskan Natives, of whom 17.2% reported tobacco use within the last 30 days.[11]

## ADOLESCENT PERCEPTIONS OF RISK OF TOBACCO USE

It is difficult to separate individual and social determinants when examining risk factors for tobacco use among youth. Adolescents are keenly cued into the social context around them and are influenced by social factors, including family, peers, and the media, each of which help shape perceptions of risk and social norms. Contextual factors associated with adolescent smoking include low socioeconomic status, low academic achievement (eg, poor grades and absenteeism), high-risk sexual behavior, and use of alcohol and other drugs.[4,12] Among girls, mothers smoking, peer smoking, and low self-esteem are associated with smoking whereas mother-daughter connectedness and higher self-seem protective, although the strength of these findings differs between white, Hispanic, and African American adolescent girls.[13] In a study of maternal smoking and children who lived with mothers who had a major depressive episode in the past year, smoking rates were increased from 5.6% if mothers neither smoked nor had a depressive episode in the last year to 15.5% for those whose mothers smoked only and 25.3% for adolescents exposed to both maternal major depressive events and maternal smoking.[14] A cross-sectional school-based survey of more than 5500 students in grades 7 through 12 revealed risk factors as well as self-reported reasons for smoking among adolescent boys and girls.[15] Among girls, risk factors for regular smoking were a history of being physically or sexually abused, violence in the home, depressive symptoms, and stressful life events. Among boys who participated in the survey, a history of physical or sexual abuse and 3 or more stressful life events were also related to increased risk of smoking. Students who were regular smokers were also asked why they smoked. Among girls, the top reasons for smoking were to help relieve stress (70.4%), being around people who smoke all the time (56.4%), cigarettes helping to keep them thin (16.2%), wanting to try and experiment (15.2%), friends encouraging them to smoke (13.3%), and wanting to be cool (3.7%). In contrast, boys who were regular smokers were less likely to identify stress (55.5%) and being around people who smoke (50.1%) or smoking to be thin (1%). Boys were more likely to state that they smoked to be cool (12.9%). In the same study, protective factors for both boys and girls were parental support and communication and participation in extracurricular activities.[15]

A body of research has attempted to understand adolescents' perceptions of risk and the social context in which tobacco use is initiated and maintained. The 2009 National Survey on Drug Use and Health queried participants about their perception of risk from a variety of behaviors. These data revealed that 65.4% of adolescent boys and 73.3% of adolescent girls perceived a great risk from smoking 1 or more packs of cigarettes per day and that risk was perceived to be higher than trying heroine once or twice, LSD once or twice, use of cocaine once a month, having 5 or more drinks of alcohol once or twice a week, or smoking marijuana once a month.[11]

Despite the high ratings of tobacco risks in recent surveys of adolescents, it is possible that many adolescents do not fully understand tobacco addiction and do not believe that they, themselves, could become addicted. A 2002 study by DiFranza and colleagues[16] suggested that approximately 20% of 679 adolescent smokers reported nicotine-dependent symptoms within 1 month of initiating smoking. A 2004 study, however, demonstrated that adolescents who smoked often believe they are less likely to become addicted than their peers who were nonsmokers.[17] Further evidence of the lack of appreciation of the addictive nature of tobacco and/or teens' overestimation of their ability to control their behaviors is abundant. For example, 56% of high school seniors who smoke contend they will still not be smoking within 5 years, but only 31% end up quitting in that time.[4] A common belief among adolescent smokers is that if they only smoke occasionally, smoke light versus regular cigarettes, or only smoke in certain situations, they are in control and will not become addicted.[18] Yet, many adolescent smokers describe using cigarettes to "feel calm" and for pleasure and emotional enjoyment, suggesting the strong role of the physiologic response to nicotine in maintaining consumption as well as the social need to "connect" with peers.[19] Thus, the addictive nature of nicotene as well as the social and emotional enjoyment of smoking plays a role in adolescents progressing from experimentation to regular tobacco use. Ever since the 1988 Surgeon General's report first outlined the effects of nicotine on promoting smoking and making it difficult to quit, there has been a huge body of research which confirms the role of nicotine dependence on adult smokers and, more recently, on adolescents.[20]

Halpern-Felsher and colleagues[18] conducted an extensive review of adolescents' and young adults' perceptions of tobacco use with special emphasis on risk perception, perceived benefits, and beliefs about addiction. They examined the popular conception of adolescent "invulnerability" that is often used to explain adolescents' decisions to engage in potentially risky behaviors. They also examined whether or not adolescents actually understand tobacco-related risks and if they can distinguish between short-term versus long-term tobacco risks. The authors conclude,

*Adolescents and young adults are aware of some of the risks involved in tobacco use and especially those consequences most stressed by public health campaigns. That is, they are aware that smoking involves a significant risk of lung cancer, heart attack and other health outcomes. However, adolescents are not aware of the full extent to which smoking is harmful, including the relative risk of smoking versus other risks, such as alcohol use or getting hit by a car. In addition, they are not as aware of the cumulative risk of tobacco use or years of life lost due to tobacco use. Importantly, adolescents are less aware and have less of an understanding of the addictive nature of tobacco use…in part because they believe they can quit at any time and therefore avoid addiction…These findings suggest that efforts to prevent or reduce tobacco use among adolescents might be more effective if they not only focus on long-term health risks but address all of adolescents' perceptions, and misperceptions, about tobacco use, including social consequences, benefits, cumulative risk, and addiction.[18(p490)]*

Recent research on risk factors for adolescent smoking and strategies for prevention have focused less on demographic characteristics or family dynamics of adolescents and instead have explored a broad range of societal influences. These include the role of the media and advertising in promoting tobacco use, easy access to tobacco products, the cost of cigarettes, and how population-level tobacco control interventions initiated over the past 20 years have affected particular population subgroups, including children and adolescents. There is consensus that depictions of tobacco in the media and movies promote smoking initiation[21] and that there is a strong relationship between tobacco marketing expenditures and tobacco consumption in the general population. In addition, there is evidence of a connection among tobacco advertising exposure, adolescent initiation of tobacco use, and progression of children and adolescents to regular tobacco use.[21] Thus, individual psychosocial risk factors, demographic characteristics, and adolescent perceptions of risk and ability to avoid addiction are best understood within the context of the physical and social environments, which help shape values, social norms, and, ultimately, tobacco-related behaviors. This suggests that the most effective methods to prevent adolescent smoking and assist in cessation are likely to be comprehensive interventions that address adolescent tobacco use simultaneously at the individual, community, and population levels.

## REDUCING YOUTH ACCESS AS AN EVIDENCE-BASED METHOD FOR PREVENTION AND CESSATION

Most experts agree that tobacco use begins as a pediatric issue. Sales to minors generate profits for the tobacco industry, tobacco merchants, and states and municipalities that reap tobacco taxes. In addition, easy access to cigarettes and other tobacco products assures a steady stream of newly addicted smokers for the tobacco industry. Minors have been prohibited from purchasing tobacco products in most states in the United States for many decades, yet historically young people under the age of 18 have had little difficulty purchasing cigarettes and tobacco products. This occurred because not all states set a minimum age of 18 for tobacco purchases and those states and municipalities that had laws prohibiting sales to minors were often lax in enforcement. For example, in 1997, it is reported that in unannounced random inspections in which a minor attempted to purchase tobacco as part of a sting operation, the minor was successful in making the purchase in as many as 72% of attempts.[22]

For more than 40 years, public health advocates around the country, including the author, have formed coalitions at the local and state levels to enact laws to prohibit tobacco sales to minors and/or insure that existing laws are enforced. The tobacco industry, in turn, has worked tirelessly with elected officials and behind the scenes to discourage changes in laws and enhanced enforcement. Health advocates also lobbied at the federal level for federal action to insure uniform minimum age for tobacco purchases in all states and assure compliance of merchants. In 1992, Congress enacted the Alcohol, Drug Abuse, and Mental Health Administration Reorganization Act (P.L. 102–321), which includes the Synar Amendment (section 1926). This historic piece of legislation is aimed at decreasing youth access to tobacco by requiring states to enact and enforce laws prohibiting the sale or distribution of tobacco products to youth under 18 years of age. To put real teeth in the legislation, states are required to conduct annual random, unannounced inspections of retail tobacco outlets and report the findings to the Secretary of Health and Human Services. The penalty for states' noncompliance in reporting is a reduction of up to 40% of that state's federal assistance for substance abuse prevention and treatment. **Fig. 2** depicts the national weighted average violation rate and shows a downward trend in retailer violation rates from 1997 to 2010.[22]

The reduction in merchant violations in response to the federal Synar Amendment corresponds to the reduction in youth smoking, suggesting that reducing minors' easy access to tobacco products is an effective policy to reduce adolescent smoking. Strategies to reduce minors' access to tobacco, however, are likely to be most effective if they are comprehensive, are multifaceted, and involve many sectors of the community committed to tobacco control. Unannounced random inspections of retail outlets and vending machines using trained youth under 18 are most effective when coupled with merchant education. In addition, coalitions of public health advocates can assist in nonenforcement compliance checks to warn noncompliant retailers and reward law-abiding retailers with public recognition. The most important element that seems to have reduced merchant violations is actively enforcing youth access laws consistently statewide.[22] Unfortunately, tobacco sales to minors persist and, in some states, up to 16.7% of merchants were found to be in violation of Synar rules in 2010. In addition, minors are resourceful in getting cigarettes and other tobacco products. Minors often get cigarettes from parents, older siblings, or peers; recruit a person over 18 to make a purchase; purchase from an unsupervised vending machine; or steal cigarettes and other tobacco products. Local ordinances that require tobacco products to be kept behind the counter discourage youth access. States with the strongest policies to limit the sale of cigarettes to minors and restrict smoking in public places have the lowest smoking rates among youth.[23] Nurses can assure that the rate of illegal sales to minors continues to decline in their own state by becoming active in their local tobacco control coalition.

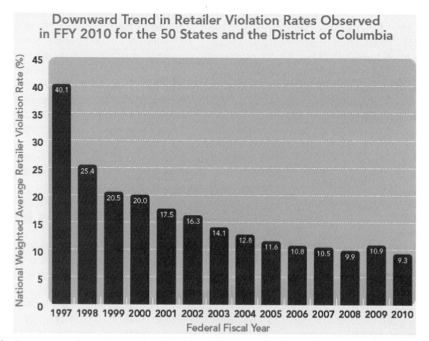

**Fig. 2.** Downward trend in retailer violation rates observed in federal fiscal year 2010 for the 50 states and the District of Columbia. (*From* Substance Abuse and Mental Health Services Administration. Fiscal year 2010 SYNAR reports: youth tobacco sales. Pub ID: SYNAR-11. Available at: http://store.samhsa.gov/shin/content//SYNAR-11/SYNAR-11.pdf. Accessed November 21, 2011.)

## COMPREHENSIVE SMOKE-FREE LEGISLATION AS AN EVIDENCE-BASED METHOD TO PREVENT ADOLESCENT TOBACCO USE AND PROMOTE CESSATION

The FCTC; the DHHS strategic plan, "Ending the Tobacco Epidemic"; and Healthy People 2020 all endorse comprehensive smoke-free policies as a way to reduce exposure to the harmful effect of secondhand smoke, encourage smokers to quit, and discourage young people from becoming smokers. Over the past 4 decades, advocates in the United States and worldwide have had increasing success in convincing policy makers to adopt comprehensive smoke-free legislation at the local, state, and, in some cases, national levels. Currently, 18 nations, 27 states, and 405 local municipalities have legislation or regulations that ban smoking in workplaces, restaurants, and bars. Many additional states and local governments have some form of restrictions on public smoking.[24] Unfortunately, the tobacco industry has continued to work vigorously at the local, state, and national levels to discourage the passage of strict smoke-free legislation.[25]

There is a wealth of research demonstrating improved health outcomes for workers in smoke-free environments as well as improvements in population health, including reductions in acute myocardial infarctions in smoke-free communities.[26] There is a growing body of research on the effects of comprehensive smoke-free policies on youth smoking behaviors. In an early study by Wakefield and colleagues,[27] the effects on adolescents of smoking restrictions at home, in the school, and in the community were investigated. Data were from a cross-sectional survey of 17,287 high school students who self-reported their smoking status. Students were classified according to 5 stages of smoking uptake with "non-susceptible non-smokers" being those who had never smoked a cigarette whereas adolescents who smoked more than 100 cigarettes in their lifetime were classified as "established smokers." The investigators concluded that smoking restrictions in a range of environments can have a protective effect on teenage smoking. Transition of teenagers through stages of taking up smoking was reduced by restrictions on home smoking and somewhat reduced by bans in public places. Smoking bans in schools had little effect unless they were strongly enforced.

Botello-Harbaum and colleagues[23] examined the relationship of youth cigarette smoking status to state-level youth access and clean indoor air laws controlling for sociodemographic characteristics and cigarette prices. Data were analyzed from the 2001–2002 Health Behavior in School-Age Children Survey and included 13,339 students in the United States. Students living in states with no or minimal restrictions during the time of the survey were more likely to be daily smokers compared with students living in states with strict regulations. Logistic regression analysis, with price and sociodemographic factors controlled, suggested that youth in states with no or limited restrictions were approximately 4 times as likely to be daily smokers than youth in states where smoking was restricted to separate or closed areas. Siegel and colleagues[28] investigated the effect of local restaurant smoking regulation on the adolescent smoking initiation process in Massachusetts. This study was conducted in 301 Massachusetts communities to assess the effects of community-level influences on smoking initiation. The study lasted 4 years and followed a cohort of 3834 youth aged 12 to 17 at baseline. Results indicated that youths living in towns with strong restaurant smoking regulations at baseline had significantly lower odds of progressing to established smoking compared with those living in towns with weak regulations.

A Canadian study of school and community characteristics and adolescent smoking concluded that schools that include tobacco prevention initiatives, prohibit smoking near school grounds, and are located in areas where tobacco prices are high have the lowest smoking rates, confirming that community-level policies affect adolescent consumption.[29] Hahn conducted a review of the health and economic outcomes of smoke-free legislation and concluded, "Studies on youth and young adults and smoke-free legislation consistently show that these laws change social norms, discouraging youth smoking uptake and established smoking."[30] Health advocates, including nurses, continue to work in coalitions across the United States and worldwide to enact comprehensive smoke-free legislation. (See description of the Nightingales, a group of nurses who have taken on the tobacco industry and are active nationwide in promoting clean air and other tobacco control policies.[31,32]) For more information about local tobacco control coalitions, contact Americans for Nonsmokers' Rights at http://no-smoke.org or your local chapter of the American Cancer Society (http://www.cancer.org), the American Lung Association (http://www.lungusa.org), the American Heart Association (http://www.heart.org/HEARTORG), or the Respiratory Health Association of Metropolitan Chicago (http://www.lungchicago.org).

## INCREASING TOBACCO TAXES AS AN EVIDENCE-BASED METHOD TO PREVENT ADOLESCENT SMOKING AND PROMOTE CESSATION

In 1999, in its report, "Curbing the Epidemic: Governments and the Economics of Tobacco Control," the World Bank leadership stated, "The most effective way to deter children from taking up smoking is to increase taxes on tobacco. High prices prevent some children and adolescents from starting and encourage those who already smoke to reduce their consumption."[33] The FCTC and DHHS strategies outlined in "Ending the Tobacco Epidemic" and in Healthy People 2020 framework all endorse raising tobacco taxes as an effective method of reducing consumption and the subsequent mortality and morbidity caused by tobacco use. Cigarettes and other tobacco products are taxed by federal, state, and local governments through excise taxes that are levied per unit (ie, per pack of cigarettes). These taxes are set by legislation and are typically collected before the point of sale from manufacturers, wholesalers, or distributors. States vary in their cigarette tax rates from a low of $0.07 a pack in South Carolina to $2.75 per pack in New York, with a national state average of $1.20.[34] The higher the state or federal tax rate, the more costly the tobacco products for the consumer. State or local sales taxes may also be levied, further raising the price. In April 2009, the largest federal cigarette excise tax increase in history went into effect, bringing the combined federal and average state excise tax for cigarettes to $2.21 per pack. This achieved the Healthy People 2010 objective of increasing combined federal and average state cigarette excise taxes to at least $2.00 per pack.[34]

There are many studies on the effect of tobacco prices and use levels. One of the landmark studies on the reduction in smoking due to increased cost per pack found that for every 10% increase in the real price of cigarettes, the number of children/youth who smoke can be expected to be reduced by 6% to 7% and the number of young adult smokers by 3.5%.[35] A 2004 study examined excise taxes and adolescent smoking behaviors in the United States using a sample of 10,981 adolescent boys and girls aged 12 to 18. Their model adjusted for age, gender, peer smoking, parental smoking, state poverty level, and possession of tobacco promotional items. It was found that higher tax rates in a state were associated with decreased odds of experimentation and also seemed protective against established smoking.[36] Cook and Carpenter[37] used data from the 1991–2005 waves of the YRBS, which contained data on more than 750,000 youths. They modeled the effects of state cigarette taxes on youth smoking controlling for survey demographics and other factors. They concluded that large state tobacco tax increases over the previous 15-year period were associated with significant reductions in smoking participation and the frequency of smoking by youths. A 2009 article found evidence of differential price elasticity for tobacco use across different adolescent groups using data from the National Longitudinal Study of Adolescent Health. The investigators suggest that individuals with low self-control or high discount rates are largely unresponsive to cigarette prices and may need policies other than taxation to help them reduce tobacco use.[38]

Awareness of cigarette tax increases among adolescents is also important in reducing consumption. A recent study was conducted in Minnesota before and after a $0.75-per-pack increase in the state cigarette tax. A survey was conducted among 3167 adolescents and young adults, which included a subsample of 781 past 30-day smokers. The investigators found that 76% of the past 30-day smokers noticed the tax increase and that being a heavier smoker, living with smokers, and having more close friends who were smokers were associated with being aware of the price increase. Among the past 30-day smokers, 24.1% reported reducing smoking because of the tax increase and 16.7% reported a quit attempt. Because fewer than half of the total participants in the survey noticed the cigarette tax increases, however, the investigators conclude that media campaigns to raise awareness of tax changes may increase their effectiveness.[39]

The tobacco industry is keenly aware that raising product prices reduces demand. Health advocates, including the author, are familiar with the overt and covert actions of the tobacco industry as well as front groups, such as retail merchants' associations and vending machine operators, all of whom regularly oppose increases in tobacco taxes. Internal documents from the major tobacco companies reveal both the tobacco industry's concern and some of the tactics they have used to thwart tobacco tax increases over the past 50 years. These documents provide further evidence of the importance of raising prices as a mechanism to reduce consumption, including consumption among youth.[40,41] Tobacco taxes are both an effective measure to reduce consumption and a rich source of revenue for cash-strapped states and municipalities. Increasing tobacco taxes can be expected to eventually decrease revenues as more and more smokers quit. States that periodically increase excise taxes to maintain revenue streams, however, can enhance both their fiscal soundness and the public's health, a win-win situation.

The International Agency for Research on Cancer recently evaluated the strengths of available evidence on the effect of tax and price policies to prevent and reduce tobacco use. Experts agreed that there was sufficient evidence of effectiveness of increased tobacco excise taxes and prices in reducing overall tobacco consumption, the prevalence of tobacco use, and the improvement of public health. There was also consensus that tobacco taxes prevent initiation and uptake of tobacco use among young people, promote cessation among current users, and lower consumption among those who continue to smoke.[42]

## TOBACCO ADVERTISING AND PROMOTION AND COUNTERADVERTISING TO REDUCE CONSUMPTION AMONG ADOLESCENTS

Cigarettes are one of the most heavily marketed products in the United States and the industry spends approximately $9.94 billion annually on cigarette advertising and promotion, which works out to $35 million per day.[43] Despite the denials of the tobacco industry, themes in tobacco advertising, promotional items, and product placements in movies have been exquisitely designed to meet the psychological needs of adolescents and young adults.[21] The 3 most heavily advertised brands in the United States—Marlboro, Camel, and Newport—are also the most popular brands with underage smokers. Adolescent boys often experience strong needs to feel and be seen as masculine, tough, and independent as well as wanting to be popular and gain peer approval. Adolescent girls also want to be popular and liked by peers and value being perceived as attractive, thin, and feminine. Many adolescents become rebellious and, as every parent and teacher knows, test the limits of adult-imposed norms. A normal developmental phenomenon of adolescence is seeking new experiences and trying new roles that help separate them from their former childhood and family roles. Adolescence is also a time when adolescents experience multiple stressors and some experience depression for the first time.[44]

Tobacco marketers often use themes that respond to adolescent psychological needs, such as popularity, peer acceptance, gender identity, rebelliousness, sensation seeking, independence, risk taking, and having fun. Other themes in tobacco advertising emphasize the stress-relieving properties of smoking or imply that smoking keeps women thin.[21] For example, a review of tobacco company marketing research indicates that youth-popular brands convey an image of smokers of those brands as popular, having fun, and being admired and well liked by peers in social situations.[45] Marlboro Man–themed marketing focuses on conveying that smokers of these brands are masculine, tough, and rugged and project an image of individualism, freedom, adventurousness, and confidence,[46] exactly what many adolescent boys would like to be. The Joe Camel campaign was designed to create the perception that Camel smokers are attractive to members of the opposite sex, "a successful ladies' man"; 61% of male smokers age 18 to 24 found Joe Camel attractive to the opposite sex.[47]

Brands targeted at women and girls, such as Newport and Virginia Slims, make associations with glamour, pleasure, smoking as sociable, and having fun. The long-running Virginia Slims campaign portrayed women as both wispy thin fashion models and also independent free thinkers. Other tobacco marketing themes that appeal to women and girls include assuaging anxieties about the dangers of smoking by promoting "light" and filter cigarettes designed especially for women and the ability of tobacco to relieve stress and provide satisfaction.[21] Recent marketing themes, which appeal to a demographic concerned about health, emphasize niche brands that are touted to be "fresh" and "all natural," despite the fact that they contain similar harmful components as other brands of cigarettes.

Evidence that children and youth increase tobacco initiation and uptake of tobacco products based on exposure to tobacco advertising is abundant. A 2003 Cochrane review assessed the effects of tobacco advertising and promotion on nonsmoking adolescents' future smoking behavior. The investigators stated, "based on the strength of association, consistency of findings, temporality of exposure and smoking behaviors observed as well as the theoretic plausibility regarding the impact of advertising, we conclude that tobacco advertising and promotion increases the likelihood that adolescents will start to smoke."[48] Longitudinal studies over the past decade have examined young people's receptivity to tobacco advertising and promotion, whether or not they have a favorite tobacco advertisement, and whether or not they have or use a cigarette promotional item as well as the amount of advertising to which they are exposed through multiple media sources in their environment. Data from these longitudinal studies also confirm a causal relationship between tobacco advertising, exposure to positive impressions of tobacco use in the media, and increased levels of tobacco initiation and continued consumption.[21,49–51]

Smoking in movies is an aspect of the social environment that has received much recent attention. Tobacco advertising was banned from television and radio in the

United States in 1969. Tobacco marketers then spent enormous amounts of advertising dollars on print media and outdoor advertising. Tobacco billboards were often concentrated in low-income, urban neighborhoods, leading to concerns of tobacco industry targeting young people and minority communities.[52–54] In 1998, the attorneys general of 46 states signed the Tobacco Master Settlement Agreement with the 4 largest tobacco companies in the United States to settle state suits to recover billions of dollars in costs associated with treating smoking-related illnesses. This legal agreement restricted billboard advertising of tobacco products and curtailed tobacco ads in magazines with substantial teen readership among other provisions.[55]

Recently approved rules under the Family Smoking Prevention and Tobacco Control Act of 2009[56] give the Food and Drug Administration authority to regulate tobacco products and will further restrict children's exposure to tobacco advertising when fully implemented in 2012.[57] One untoward effect of the Master Settlement Agreement, however, was that tobacco companies shifted their tobacco advertising and promotion dollars to venues not covered by the settlement agreement, such as discounting of cigarettes, increased point-of-purchase advertising, and product placements in motion pictures. Tobacco companies pay to have their products prominently displayed in the movies and have their products handled and smoked by popular actors. Product placements are not restricted to adult-targeted films and are equally likely to appear in movies rated PG-13.

Exposure to on-screen smoking in movies increases the probability that youth start smoking. Young people who are heavily exposed to on-screen smoking are approximately 2 to 3 times more likely to begin smoking than youths who are lightly exposed.[21] A similar but smaller effect exists for young adults.[58] Studies using content analysis have documented that smoking is portrayed in approximately 87% of movies produced from 1988 to 1997[59] and in 77% of movies in 2004.[60] Smoking in top-grossing films has been studied longitudinally from 1991 to 2009. The number of tobacco incidents depicted in the movies during this time peaked in 2005 and then progressively declined. For example, top-grossing movies in 2009 contained only approximately half as many on-screen smoking incidents as observed in 2005.[61] The decline in tobacco incidents in movies can be attributed to aggressive campaigns by tobacco control advocates to put pressure on the Motion Picture Association of America, movie studios, and movie stars. Several major studios adopted practices, which they claim will reduce tobacco incidents, and in 2008, 6 major movie studios said they would place antismoking public service announcements on DVDs of all movies with youth ratings that depict smoking. These antismoking messages do not appear, however, when youth-rated movies are shown in theaters.

In 2009, the WHO issued new film policy guidelines suggesting that on-screen tobacco promotion in movies should trigger adult ratings of films and strong antitobacco spots in theaters, on DVDs, and on cable, satellite, and other channels.[62] Nurses and others who are interested in working to decrease the smoking incidents in movies and rate movies with incidents of positive portrayal of tobacco rated as "R" may explore the Smoke Free Movies project begun in 2001, at the University of California, San Francisco (see http://smokefreemovies.ucsf.edu/problem/moviessell. html). Unfortunately, in countries in the developing world, tobacco companies still use multiple media sources, including movie theaters, as venues to advertise tobacco products to youth.

Mass media exerts tremendous power in our wired and socially connected society and adolescents are particularly susceptible to media influences. An important piece of a comprehensive tobacco control program is a strong countermarketing program. Tobacco countermarketing is defined as the use of commercial marketing tactics to reduce the prevalence of tobacco use. Countermarketing attempts to counter pro-tobacco influence and increase prohealth messages. In the case of adolescents, the goal of countermarketing is to directly challenge the false messages promulgated by the tobacco industry with countermessages that change attitudes and social norms to decrease the likelihood that children and young people will find tobacco use attractive. An example of an effective countermarketing initiative is the American Legacy Foundation's Truth Campaign. The Truth Campaign is the largest national youth-focused antitobacco education campaign ever. It is designed to engage teens by exposing Big Tobacco's marketing and manufacturing practices as well as high-lighting the toll of tobacco in relevant and innovative ways.[63] The Truth Campaign enlists young people to create countermarketing advertisements that are edgy and appealing to the rebelliousness of youth. Memorable countermarketing ads include the famous parody of the Marlboro Man riding up on horseback while smoking through his tracheotomy. Another is the dramatic depiction of young people delivering body bags to tobacco companies. These short videos have been used extensively as public service announcements and in media-based antitobacco campaigns. This initiative is funded by the Tobacco Master Settlement Agreement.

Other examples of countermarketing are included in many of the provisions mandated by the Family Smoking Prevention and Tobacco Control Act of 2009, which gave the Food and Drug Administration comprehensive authority to regulate tobacco products. These new regulations are aimed at countering tobacco industry marketing, prohibiting all tobacco brand sponsorships of sporting and entertainment events, restricting vending machines and self-service displays to adult-only facilities, and ending the misleading labeling of cigarettes, which use the words "light," "mild," and "low tar" to imply that some cigarettes may be less harmful. Finally, graphic warning labels will be put in place on the top half of both the front and back of cigarette packs depicting diseases lungs, a smoker with a tracheotomy hole, and a person lying in a coffin. Each of these labels directly counters tobacco company messaging.[57] As of this writing, the tobacco industry is suing the Food and Drug Administration to stall implementation of these countermarketing initiatives.

## SCHOOL-BASED SMOKING PREVENTION PROGRAMS

Many elementary and high schools include education about the risks of tobacco use and messages to avoid tobacco and drugs as part of their health or science curricula. School nurses are committed to health promotion and often provide classroom education on tobacco use avoidance. The Drug Abuse Resistance Education (D.A.R.E.) program was popular for many years and implemented widely in the United States. Selected schools have participated in a variety of organized school-based tobacco prevention programs developed by researchers over the past 30 years. Meta-analyses of school-based prevention programs have used various criteria and have had conflicting results. For example, Glantz and Mandel concluded that most school-based prevention programs do not work.[64]

A recent review of the long-term promise of the effectiveness of school-based prevention programs was conducted by Flay as part of the National Academy of Science's *Ending the Tobacco Problem: A Blueprint for the Nation*.[65] The purpose was to determine what long-term effects the nation might expect if successful evidence-based school and community prevention programs were to be adopted nationwide.[65] For the review, published studies were categorized as category 1 if they included 15 or more sessions, preferably including some high school sessions, and had demonstrated short-term, medium-term, and/or long-term effects. These programs could be school based or school plus community/mass media programs. The outcome measure used was percent relative reduction in smoking at follow-up. Programs reviewed included the Tobacco and Alcohol Prevention Project, Life Skills Training, and Project SHOUT. These programs used a variety of social influence approaches: practicing refusal and other assertion skills, information about the health and social consequences of tobacco use, and, in the case of Project Shout, participation in community action projects designed to mobilize young people as antitobacco activists. Results from category 1 school-based programs revealed significant medium-term effects at grades 10 and 12. This means that there was approximately a 27% reduction in smoking initiation among those who participated.[65]

School-based plus community/mass media programs were also reviewed, including the North Karelia Project in Finland, the Class of 1989 Study, the Midwestern Prevention Project, and the Vermont Mass Media Project. These programs were found to have higher reductions in smoking initiation of approximately 40% at the end of the program but over time reductions decayed to approximately 31%. It was concluded that the delivery of multiple modalities in the community, along with school programs, is likely to increase effectiveness compared with school-only programs.[65]

The review also included several programs with exceptional promise or which could provide other insights about possible program effectiveness in reducing smoking onset if prevention programs were widely implemented. These programs included the Adolescent Alcohol Prevention Trial, Towards No Tobacco, Know Your Body, and the Good Behavior Game. Even though these programs were varied, they demonstrated a 27.2% short-term effect and a 39.1% medium-term effect, usually in the eighth or ninth grade. The range of smoking initiation reduction, however, was large, ranging from 12% to 49% in the short term and 26% to 73% for medium term. The review also identified programs that are ineffective, such as D.A.R.E. and Hutchinson Smoking Prevention Project programs, both of which are not recommended. Flay concludes with recommendations. Based on the literature reviewed and the assumption of full implementation of the most effective, comprehensive school plus community/mass media programs, it might be possible to reduce smoking initiation by age 25 by as much as 26%. Flay hypothesizes, however, that in real-life situations, school plus community/mass media programs could be expected to reduce tobacco use by age 25 by approximately 20%.[65] Nurses can identify evidence-based interventions likely to be effective and support their implementation in schools.

## EVIDENCE-BASED TOBACCO CESSATION PROGRAMS FOR ADOLESCENTS

Cigarette smoking among adolescents is a multidimensional behavior affected by the interaction of biologic, psychosocial, and environmental determinants. Quitting smoking is also complex due to the addictive nature of nicotine and the developmental level of adolescents, which is often characterized by immature psychosocial capacities, poor impulse control, and a lack of well-developed coping skills. Similar to adults, adolescents who smoke often state they wish to quit and almost half of adolescents who smoked in the previous year state they made a quit attempt.[66] The majority of these quit attempts apparently occur without the support of evidence-based tobacco cessation programs.[67]

Despite the need for effective interventions to aid adolescents in quitting, the number of published studies of tobacco cessation treatments that meet criteria for systematic evaluation is small. A systematic review of youth cessation interventions that captured studies conducted before 2006 was published by Grimshaw and

Stanton and updated in 2009.[68] A meta-analysis of teen cigarette smoking cessation was published in 2006 by Sussman and colleagues,[69] and Curry and colleagues reviewed youth tobacco cessation interventions in 2009.[70] Currently, the Robert Wood Johnson Foundation, with additional support from the National Cancer Institute and the Centers for Disease Control and Prevention, is funding a 3-phase initiative to identify best practices in tobacco cessation for youth. Phase 1 is the identification of a national sample of existing community-based tobacco-cessation programs for youth,[67] and phase 2 will describe the program design and implementation to assist in identifying best practices within existing cessation programs.[71]

In each of these review articles, the conceptual framework for youth cessation programs was categorized for ease of analysis. The most common conceptual frameworks included Prochaska's Transtheoretical Model of the five stages of change[72]; social influence models, which emphasize social interactions and peer relationships that can support or undermine cessation efforts and/or counter tobacco industry influences; and motivational enhancement models that attempt to increase reasons for youth to quit and address their concerns and ambivalence about tobacco use cessation. Other models include cognitive behavioral therapy (CBT), which focuses on learning coping skills and problem-solving strategies for understanding and, hopefully, disrupting patterns of tobacco use. CBT is also designed to help adolescents deal with tobacco use cravings, manage stressful situations, and resist social pressures to smoke.[70] At the time these reviews were completed, pharmacologic interventions were not widespread.

Many interventions targeted at helping adolescents to quit are challenged by difficulties in recruiting sufficient numbers of youth to meet statistical criteria for effect size. Adolescents are often reluctant to join organized programs, even when these programs are conveniently offered in their own school setting. Programs offered in schools often have difficulty negotiating with administrators for time away from class and/or gaining approvals for parental consent. In addition, as in many longitudinal research designs, it is difficult to maintain cohorts and complete follow-up due to high attrition in longitudinal studies.[70] Published studies of adolescent-targeted cessation programs frequently have serious methodologic issues. These include a lack of a standard methodology of how to measure baseline smoking, lack of a standardized measure for quitting/abstinence, and no standardized time to follow-up to see if abstinence is maintained. Other methodologic problems encountered are lack of full description of the program and concerns about program fidelity (ie, if the program actually offered as planned). Therefore, each of the existing systematic reviews and meta-analyses used slightly different inclusion and exclusion criteria.[70]

The Sussman and colleagues[69] meta-analysis of teen cigarette smoking cessation examined 48 published studies and found higher quit rates in programs that included motivational enhancement, CBT techniques, and social influence approaches. They also suggest higher quit rates in school-based clinic and classroom modalities and in those programs consisting of at least 5 quit sessions. Some effects were maintained at short term (1 year or less) or longer term (longer than 1 year). They concluded that much more teen cessation research is needed but teen smoking cessation programming can be effective. The Grimshaw and Stanton systematic review identified 24 trials involving more than 5000 young people who met inclusion criteria. They found that many interventions combined theoretic frameworks but most used some form of motivational enhancements combined with psychological support, such as CBT and use of the Transtheoretical Model. They stated that complex approaches show promise and some demonstrated persistence of abstinence at 30 days or continuous abstinence at 6 months and those interventions incorporating elements sensitive to stages of change, motivational enhancement, and CBT were most promising. The conclusion, however, was that there is not yet sufficient evidence to recommend wide-spread implementation of any one model.[68]

Curry and colleagues[70] summarized findings from existing systematic reviews and meta-analyses and identified additional published studies to add to the existing data-base. These researchers included exploration of the effect of the setting, such as schools versus health care settings, and also looked at several innovative channels for delivering cessation, such as telephone counseling and other technology-based platforms, such as Web-based programs. In addition, they identified 2 studies using either bupropion or nicotine replacement. They also discuss the potential impact of mandatory treatment because some programs include young people who are mandated to participate because they are underage smokers who got caught and were "sentenced" to cessation programs. They conclude

*A sufficient number of good quality youth cessation intervention studies now exist to provide evidence-based recommendations based on meta-analyses. We can say confidently that behavioral interventions increase the chances of youth smokers achieving successful cessation...Motivational enhancements and cognitive behavioral approaches appear to be efficacious with youth. Currently, there is no evidence that nicotine replacement treatment aids youth cessation...Innovative studies have been compromised by recruiting sufficient number of youth, obtaining approval for waivers of parental consent and high attri-tion in longitudinal data collection.*[70(p245-6)]

A description of the state of the art in tobacco cessation programs for youth is not complete without including the preliminary findings of Curry and colleagues[67] of their national survey of existing programs. Researchers used key informant interview snowball sampling methods to profile 591 programs that had provided treatment to more than 36,000 youths in the previous year. They categorized programs by geographic area, setting, and type of program offered and found considerable homogeneity among programs. The typical program was multisession and offered in a school but served few numbers of young people each year. Consistent with other research findings, most programs included cognitive behavioral components and externally developed materials. Some of the most popular programs were the American Lung Association's Not On Tobacco program, which has been categorized as an evidence-based program by the Substance Abuse and Mental Health Services Administration. They also found programs often had a provision for mandatory participation but this was not a large percentage of participants. Most evaluations were performed internally and programs operated on a limited budget. A disturbing finding was the inverse association between the need for cessation programming on the basis of trends in smoking prevalence and program availability. For example, there was less availability of cessation programs in nonurban counties and counties with low socioeconomic status, even though smoking rates are higher in these areas. The investigators conclude that replicable programs exist in communities across the United States and that rigorous program evaluations are needed to inform best practices for tobacco cessation in youth.[67] The national evaluation of community-based cessation programs is continuing in phase 2.[71]

Recently, increasing attention has been focused on the potential of Web-based interventions for smoking cessation among adolescents. This makes sense because children and adolescents are masters of cell phones, iPods, iPads, and all manner of portable technology to stay connected. A systematic review conducted by Hutton and colleagues[73] identified 5 randomized controlled trials of Web-based interventions among adolescents. They report that these studies demonstrated mixed results with insufficient evidence to support their efficacy.

## SUMMARY AND RECOMMENDATIONS

Tobacco use among adolescents is declining in the United States but remains a major public health problem in the United States and globally. The Healthy People 2020 model of determinants of health is useful in understanding the complex interaction of factors that help explain adolescent smoking-related behaviors. Biology and genetics, individual behavior, social environment, physical environment, and access to health care and evidence-based programs all affect tobacco use among youth. The WHO, DHHS, and Centers for Disease Control and Prevention plus many public health experts recommend a variety of evidence-based interventions that can be implemented at the individual, community, population, and global levels. Participation in organized school or community prevention programs has the potential to enhance an adolescent's probability of avoiding future tobacco use if the best programs are fully implemented. Participation in evidence-based cessation programs increases the odds of successful quitting but additional strategies are needed to improve quit rates and make effective programs much more widely available for adolescents who smoke. Program components likely to increase resistance to tobacco or success in quitting have been identified, such as cognitive behavioral techniques and strategies to address influences in the social environment that encourage tobacco use. Changing social norms about tobacco is key to creating a world free of tobacco. Many of the most effective methods for keeping adolescents tobacco-free are interventions implemented at the community and population levels, such as youth access laws, increasing the price of tobacco, smoke-free legislation, restrictions on tobacco advertising and promotion, and changing a media culture that often encourages tobacco use. Counteradvertising, especially messaging that appeals to youths' rebelliousness, is also promising. Additional research is needed that links population-based interventions, such as mass media campaigns, tobacco taxes, maintaining smoke-free environments, and restricting tobacco advertising targeted at youth with school and community evidence-based prevention and cessation programs to evaluate possible synergistic effects. Nurses are well positioned to take leadership roles in health care settings, schools, and their own communities as well as at the state, national, and global levels in advocating for policies that prevent adolescent tobacco use and the subsequent burden of disease in future populations.

## REFERENCES

1. World Health Organization. World No Tobacco Day 2011. Available at: http://www.who.int/tobacco/wntd/2011/flyer/en/index.html. Accessed November 21, 2011.
2. CDC. Smoking-attributable mortality, years of potential life lost, and productivity losses—United States, 2000-2004. MMWR Morb Mortal Wkly Rep 2008;57(45): 1226–8.
3. Results from the 2008 National Survey on Drug Use and Health: National Findings (Office of Applied Studies, NSDUH Series H-36, HHS Publication No. SMA 09–4434). Rockville (MD): Substance Abuse and Mental Health Services Administration; 2009.
4. U.S. Department of Health and Human Services, Office of the Surgeon General. Preventing tobacco use among young people: a report of the Surgeon General. Atlanta (GA): US Department of Health and Human Services, CDC; 1994.

Available at: http://www.cdc.gov/tobacco/data_statistics/sgr/1994/index.htm. Accessed November 21, 2011.

5. U.S. v. Philip Morris USA, Inc., et al. No. 99–CV02496GK (U.S. Dist. Ct., D.C.), Final Opinion, August 17, 2006. Available at: http://www.tobaccofreekids.org/content/what_we_do/industry_watch/doj/FinalOpinionSummary.pdf. Accessed November 21, 2011.

6. World Health Organization. Framework Convention on Tobacco Control. Available at: http://www.who.int/fctc/en. Accessed November 21, 2011.

7. U.S. Department of Health and Human Services. Ending the tobacco epidemic: a tobacco control strategic action plan. Available at: http://www.hhs.gov/ash/initiatives/tobacco/tobaccostrategicplan2010.pdf. Accessed November 21, 2011.

8. U.S. Department of Health and Human Services. Office of Disease Prevention and Health Promotion. Healthy People 2020. Available at: http://www.healthypeople.gov/2020/default.aspx. Accessed November 21, 2011.

9. Centers for Disease Control and Prevention. Cigarette use among high school students—United States, 1991-2009. MMWR Morb Mortal Wkly Rep 2010; 59(27):797–801.

10. Youth Risk Behavior Survey. Available at: http://www.cdc.gov/healthyyouth/yrbs/pdf/us_tobacco_trend_yrbs.pdf. Accessed November 21, 2011.

11. Substance Abuse and Mental Health Services Administration, Office of Applied Studies. The NSDUH Report: perceptions of risk from substance use among adolescents. Rockville (MD). Pub ID: NSDUH09–1126. Available at: http://oas.samhsa.gov/2k9/158/158RiskPerceptionHTML.pdf. 2009. Accessed November 21, 2011.

12. U.S. Department of Health and Human Services, Office of the Surgeon General. Reducing tobacco use: a report of the Surgeon General. Atlanta (GA): US Department of Health and Human Services, CDC; 2000. Available at: http://www.surgeongeneral.gov/library/tobacco_use/index.html. Accessed November 21, 2011.

13. Faucher MA. Factors that influence smoking in adolescent girls. J Midwifery Womens Health 2003;48(3):199–205.

14. Substance Abuse and Mental Health Services Administration, Office of Applied Studies. The NSDUH Report: adolescent smoking and maternal risk factors. Rockville, MD. Pub id: NSDUH10–0507. 2010. Available at: http://www.oas.samhsa.gov/2k10/166/166SmokingMoms.htm. Accessed November 21, 2011.

15. Simantov E, Schoen C, Klein J. Health-compromising behaviors: why do adolescents smoke or drink? Identifying underlying risk and protective factors. Arch Pediatr Adolesc Med 2000;154(10):1025–33.

16. DiFranza J, Savageau J, Rigotti N, et al. Development of symptoms of tobacco dependence in youths: thirty month follow up data from the DANDY study. Tob Control 2002;11(3):228–35.

17. Halpern-Felsher B, Biehl M, Kropp R, et al. Perceived risks and benefits of smoking: differences among adolescents with different smoking experiences and intentions. Prev Med 2004;39(3):559–67.

18. Halpern-Felsher B, Ramos M, Cornell J. Appendix E. Adolescents' and young adults' perceptions of tobacco use: a review and critique of the current literature. In: Institute of Medicine, editor. Ending the tobacco problem: a blueprint for the Nation. Washington, DC: National Academies Press; 2007. p. 490.

19. Johnson J, Bottorff J, Moffat B, et al. Tobacco dependence: adolescents' perspectives on the need to smoke. Soc Sci Med 2003;56(7):1481–92.

20. Institute of Medicine. Ending the tobacco problem: a blueprint for the nation. Chapter 2. Factors perpetuating the tobacco problem. Washington, DC: The National Academies Press; 2007.

21. Davis R, Gilpin E, Loken B, et al, editors. Monograph 19—the role of the media in reporting and reducing tobacco use. In National Cancer Institute Tobacco Control Monograph Series: Public Health Issues in Smoking and Tobacco Use Control. 2008. Available at: http://cancercontrol.cancer.gov/tcrb/monographs. Accessed November 21, 2011.

22. Substance Abuse and Mental Health Services Administration. (2011). Fiscal year 2010 SYNAR reports: youth tobacco sales. Pub ID: SYNAR-11. Available at: http://store.samhsa.gov/shin/content//SYNAR-11/SYNAR-11.pdf. Accessed November 21, 2011.

23. Botello-Harbaum M, Haynie D, Iannotti R, et al. Tobacco control policy and adolescent cigarette smoking status in the United States. Nicotine Tob Res 2009;11(7):875–85.

24. American Lung Association. State of tobacco control 2010. Available at: http://www.stateoftobaccocontrol.org. Accessed November 21, 2011.

25. Campaign for Tobacco Free Kids. Fact sheets on secondhand smoke. Available at: http://www.tobaccofreekids.org/facts_issues/fact_sheets/policies/secondhand_smoke. Accessed November 21, 2011.

26. Myers D, Neuberger J, He J. Cardiovascular effect of bans on smoking in public places: a systematic review & meta-analysis. J Am Coll Cardiol 2009;54(14):1249–55.

27. Wakefield M, Chaloupka F, Kaufman N, et al. Effect of restrictions on smoking at home, at school, and in public places on teenage smoking: cross sectional study. BMJ 2000;321(7257):333–7.

28. Siegel M, Albers A, Cheng D, et al. Local restaurant smoking regulations and the adolescent smoking initiation process: results of a multilevel contextual analysis among Massachusetts youth. Arch Pediatr Adolesc Med 2008;162(5):477–83.

29. Lovatto C, Zeisser C, Campbell S, et al. Adolescent smoking: effect of school and community characteristics. Am J Prev Med 2010;39(6):507–14.

30. Hahn E. Smokefree legislation: a review of health and economic outcomes research. Am J Prev Med 2010;39(6 Suppl 1):S66–76.

31. Mason D, Leavitt J, Chaffee M. Policy and politics in nursing and health care. 6th edition. St Louis (MO): Elsevier-Saunders; 2012.

32. The Nightingales. Available at: http://nightingalesnurses.org. Accessed November 21, 2011.

33. Jha P, Chaloupka FJ. Curbing the epidemic: governments and the economics of tobacco control. Washington, DC: World Bank; 1999. Available at: http://www-wds.worldbank.org/external/default/WDSContentServer/IW3P/IB/2000/08/02/000094946_99092312090116/Rendered/PDF/multi_page.pdf. Accessed November 21, 2011.

34. CDC. Federal and state cigarette excise taxes—United States, 1995–2009. MMWR Morb Mortal Wkly Rep 2009;58(19):524–7.

35. Chaloupka F. Macro-social influences: the effects of prices and tobacco control policies on the demand for tobacco products. Nicotine Tob Res 1999;1(1):S105–9.

36. Thomson C, Fisher L, Winickoff J, et al. State tobacco excise taxes and adolescent smoking behaviors in the United States. J Public Health Manag Pract 2004;10(6):490–6.

37. Carpenter C, Cook P. Cigarette taxes and youth smoking: new evidence from national, state and local Youth Risk Behavior Surveys. J Health Econ 2008;27(2):287–99.

38. Fletcher J, Deb P, Sindelar J. NBER Working Paper No. 15130: tobacco use, taxation and self control in adolescence. Issued in July 2009. Washington, DC: National Bureau of Economic Research; 2009. Available at: http://www.nber.org/papers/w15130.pdf?new_window=1. Accessed November 21, 2011.
39. Choi T, Toomey T, Chen V, et al. Awareness and reported consequences of a cigarette tax increase among older adolescents and young adults. Am J Health Promot 2011;25(6):379–86.
40. Campaign for Tobacco-Free Kids. Higher tobacco taxes reduce tobacco use. Available at: http://www.tobaccofreekids.org/facts_issues/fact_sheets/policies/tax/us_state_local. Accessed November 21, 2011.
41. Chaloupka F, Cummings K, Morley C, et al. Tax, price and cigarette smoking: evidence from the tobacco documents and implications for tobacco company marketing strategies. Tob Control 2002;11(Suppl 1):i62–72.
42. Chaloupka F, Straif K, Leon M. Effectiveness of tax and price policies in tobacco control. Tob Control 2011;20(3):235–8.
43. Federal Trade Commission. FTC releases reports on cigarette and smokeless tobacco advertising and promotion: amount spent declines for cigarettes, increases for smokeless tobacco in 2007 and 2008. 2011. Available at: http://www.ftc.gov/opa/2011/07/tobacco.shtm. Accessed November 21, 2011.
44. Steinberg L. Adolescence. 8th edition. New York: McGraw-Hill; 2008.
45. Legacy Tobacco Documents Library. 8102 Young smokers prevalence, trends, implications, and related demographics. Bates No. 1000390803/0855. 1981. Available at: http://legacy.library.ucsf.edu/tid/ftu74e00. Accessed November 21, 2011.
46. Legacy Tobacco Documents Library. Marlboro/Camel consumer research. Bates No. 2071581345/1365. 1991. Available at: http://legacy.library.ucsf.edu/tid/vio26c00. Accessed November 21, 2011.
47. Legacy Tobacco Documents Library, Reynolds RJ. "Smooth character" campaign. Bates No. 507244164/4184. 1989. Available at: http://legacy.library.ucsf.edu/tid/lpi54d00. Accessed November 21, 2011.
48. Lovato C, Linn G, Stead L, et al. Impact of tobacco advertising and promotion on increasing adolescent smoking behaviours. Cochrane Database Syst Rev 2003; 4:CD003439. DOI:10.1002/14651858.CD003439.
49. Biener L, Siegel M. Tobacco marketing and adolescent smoking: more support for a causal inference. Am J Public Health 2000;90(3):407–11.
50. Choi W, Ahluwalia J, Harris K, et al. Progression to established smoking: the influence of tobacco marketing. Am J Prev Med 2002;22(4):228–33.
51. Gilpin E, White M, Messer K, et al. Receptivity to tobacco advertising and promotions among young adolescents as a predictor of established smoking in young adulthood. Am J Public Health 2007;97(8):1489–95.
52. Hackbarth D, Silvestri B, Cosper W. Tobacco and alcohol billboards in 50 Chicago neighborhoods: market segmentation to sell dangerous products to the poor. J Public Health Policy 1995;16(2):213–30.
53. Hackbarth D, Schnopp-Wyatt D. Tobacco advertising restrictions as primary prevention for childhood nicotine addiction. J Addict Nurs 1997;9(3):112–7.
54. Hackbarth D, Schnopp-Wyatt D, Katz D, et al. Collaborative research and action to control the geographic placement of outdoor advertising of age restricted products in Chicago. Public Health Rep 2001;116:558–67.
55. National Association of Attorneys General. Available at: http://naag.org/tobacco.php. Accessed November 21, 2011.
56. Family Smoking Prevention and Tobacco Control Act of 2009. Available at: http://www.govtrack.us/congress/bill.xpd?bill=h111-1256. Accessed November 21, 2011.

57. Food and Drug Administration. Available at: http://www.fda.gov/Food/Food Safety/FSMA/ucm237092.htm. Accessed November 21, 2011.
58. Song A, Ling P, Nielands T, et al. Smoking in movies and increased smoking among young adults. Am J Prev Med 2007;33:396–403.
59. Dalton M, Tickle J, Sargent JD, et al. The incidence and context of tobacco use in popular movies from 1988 to 1997. Prev Med 2002;34(5):516–23.
60. Worth K, Tanski S, Saragent J. Trends in top box office movie tobacco use, 1996-2004. First Look Report. Washington, DC: American Legacy Foundation; 2006.
61. CDC. Smoking in top-grossing movies—United States, 1991-2009. MMWR Morb Mortal Wkly Rep 2010;59(32):1014–7.
62. Monograph: smoke-free movies: from evidence to action. WHO; 2009. Available at: http://whqlibdoc.who.int/publications/2009/9789241597937_eng.pdf. Accessed November 21, 2011.
63. American Legacy Foundation Truth Campaign. Available at: http://www.thetruth.com. Accessed November 21, 2011.
64. Glantz S, Mandel L. Since school-based tobacco prevention programs do not work, what should we do? J Adolesc Health 2005;36(3):157–9.
65. Flay B. Appendix D: the long-term promise of effective school-based smoking prevention programs. In: Institute of Medicine, editor. Ending the tobacco problem: a blueprint for the nation. Washington, DC: The National Academies Press; 2007. p. 449–77.
66. CDC. Tobacco Use and United States Students. Available at: http://www.cdc.gov/healthyyouth/yrbs/pdf/us_tobacco_combo.pdf. Accessed November 21, 2011.
67. Curry S, Emery S, Sporer A, et al. A national survey of tobacco cessation programs for youths. Am J Public Health 2007;97(1):171–7.
68. Grimshaw G, Stanton A. Tobacco cessation interventions for young people. Cochrane Database Syst Rev 2009;1:CD003289. DOI:10.1002/14651858.CD003289.pub4.
69. Sussman S, Sun P, Dent C. A meta-analysis of teen cigarette smoking cessation. Health Psychol 2006;25(5):549–57.
70. Curry S, Mermelstein R, Sporer A. Therapy for specific problems: youth tobacco cessation. Annu Rev Psychol 2009;60:229–55.
71. Curry S, Mermelstein R, Sporer A, et al. A national evaluation of community-based youth cessation programs: design and implementation. Eval Rev 2010; 34(6):487–512.
72. Prochaska J, DiClemente C, Norcross J. In search of how people change: applications to the addictive behaviors. Am Psychol 1992;47:1102–14.
73. Hutton H, Wilson L, Apelberg B, et al. A systematic review of randomized controlled trials: web-based interventions for smoking cessation among adolescents, college students, and adults. Nicotine Tob Res 2011;13(4):227–38.

# Water Pipe Smoking Among the Young: The Rebirth of an Old Tradition

Virginia Hill Rice, PhD, RN, CNS

## KEYWORDS

- Water pipe smoking • Hookah • Tobacco use • Youth
- Adolescents • Health outcomes

Tobacco use, primarily cigarette smoking is the second most preventable cause of death and disability in the world.[1] In the United States (U.S.), it is the number one most preventable cause, being responsible for about 1 in 5 (or approximately 443,000) deaths each year.[2] An estimated 49,000 of these deaths are related to secondhand smoke exposure.[3] Cigarette smoking costs this nation more than $193 billion annually (ie, $97 billion for lost productivity and $96,000 in health care expenditures) with additional costs for secondhand smoke health problems at more than $10 million.[4] On average, male smokers shorten their lives by 13.2 years, and female smokers lose 14.5 years.[5] In addition to the burden of cigarette smoking is the growing use of other tobacco products, such as chewing tobacco, cigars, moist and dry snuff, and water pipe smoking.[6]

## WATER PIPE (HOOKAH) SMOKING

Water pipe smoking (WPS), also known as the hookah, shisha, narghile, arghile, and hubble bubble (depending on where you are in the world), is a 500-year-old form of tobacco use historically engaged in by older men in the Middle East, North Africa, and Asia. The water pipe (WP) is a symbol of social sharing and cultural identity in the Middle East.[7] Since the early 1990s, there has been a significant increase in its use around the world[8] and in the United States.[9,10] Wolfram and colleagues[11] reported that more than 100 million people worldwide smoke hookahs daily.

---

Research for our study of tobacco use in Arab American youth was funded by the Eunice Kennedy Shriver National Institute of Child Health and Human Development (HD37498-RO1).
Adult Health, Wayne State University College of Nursing and Karmanos Cancer Center, 366 Cohn Building, 5557 Cass Avenue, Detroit, MI 4820, USA
*E-mail address:* vrice@wayne.edu

Nurs Clin N Am 47 (2012) 141–148
doi:10.1016/j.cnur.2011.10.011
0029-6465/12/$ – see front matter © 2012 Elsevier Inc. All rights reserved.

## THE WATER PIPE

The WP operates by water filtration and indirect heat (**Fig. 1**). It has 4 fundamental parts: (1) a head where a special tobacco is placed and heated (usually by charcoal or burning embers); (2) a bowl or smoke chamber, which is partially filled with water; (3) a pipe or body connecting the head to the bowl by a tube that carries the smoke downward into the water; and (4) a hose with a mouthpiece through which the smoke is drawn from the bowl. As the smoker inhales, the tobacco smoke is sucked downward into the bowl and then bubbles up through the water into the air of the smoke chamber, and then through the hose to the smoker. The water cools the smoke and filters out a very small amount of tars and particulates[12] and about 5% of the nicotine.[13] In the Arab world, people see the hookah as representing their past and their traditions.

Social smoking is done with a single or double hose, and sometimes a triple or quadruple hose in parties or small get-togethers. When the smoker is finished, either the hose is placed back on the table signifying that it is available or it is handed from one user to the next. If on the table, the hose must be folded back on itself so that the mouthpiece is not pointing at another recipient. Smoking the WP is a "ceremonial" activity governed by rules for each stage of the preparing, lighting, sharing, and smoking process.[14] WP units come in a variety of materials (eg, glass, ceramic, metal), designs, and sizes. There are hundreds of Web sites to learn about WPS and its history and to purchase its elements for personal use (eg, http://sacrednarghile.com/en/index.php).

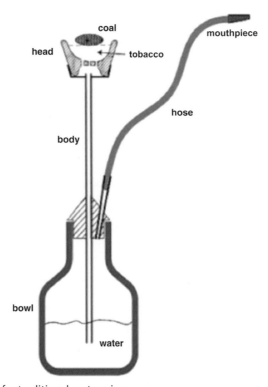

**Fig. 1.** Diagram of a traditional water pipe.

## WATER PIPE SMOKING PREVALENCE

Global Tobacco Youth Survey data from nationally representative samples of students (13–15 years) from 7 countries in the Middle East were collected between 2001 and 2005. The results confirmed that boys are significantly more likely than girls to smoke cigarettes or to use the shisha (water pipe). Students had higher rates of tobacco use than adults in Bahrain, Oman, and the United Arab Emirates. For both boys and girls, WPS rates were higher than cigarette smoking rates in almost all of the countries.[15] Akl and his colleagues[16] reviewed 38 studies; only 4 were national surveys, the rest evaluated specific populations. The highest prevalence of current WPS was among adolescent high school students in the Arabic Gulf region (9%–16%), Estonia (21%), and Lebanon (25%). Current WPS, defined as used in the past 30 days, by university students was high in the Arabic Gulf region (6%), the United Kingdom (8%), the United States (10%), Syria (15%), Lebanon (28%), and Pakistan (33%). Current WPS for adults included those in Pakistan (6%), the Arabic Gulf region (4%–12%), Australia (11% in Arab-speaking adults), and Lebanon (15%). The World Health Organization's (WHO) highest rates for adults in 2008 were in Jordan (61.7%) and Tunisia (51%), followed by the Syrian Arab Republic (42%).[17]

Major reasons for the growing popularity worldwide of the WP include migrations of people from regions where WPS is commonly used,[18] the "new" molasses-flavored and fruit-flavored tobacco mixes (eg, maassel),[8] public restaurants and cafes that host WPS, and the adoption of WPS as youths.[19–21] In the Middle East, limited research has documented WPS because of its long standing as a social tradition,[22,23] and the unsubstantiated belief that it is less harmful than cigarettes or other tobacco products.[21,24] WHO and the American Lung Association study teams both indicated a need for more thorough investigations of the water pipe and its risks and health effects wherever it was being used.[8,9] A country that is showing increased WPS is the United States.[9,10]

### Arab Americans

Although there are no national or even regional water pipe smoking databases in the United States, the American Lung Association[9] has labeled it "…the first new tobacco trend of the 21st century"[9] and has linked its use to the growing numbers of those with a Middle Eastern heritage. This population first came to the American auto industry in small working groups at the turn of the last century; the number of Middle Eastern immigrants has grown dramatically in the past 50 to 60 years because of wars, religious conflicts, and political struggles. Today, more than 4 million claim an Arab American heritage.[25] Most, around 62%, originated from the region of the Levant, which includes Syria, Lebanon, Palestine/Israel, Egypt, and Lebanon. The rest are from Jordan, Iraq, Libya, Morocco, and many other small Arab nations. Arab Americans live in all 50 states and Washington, DC; 94% reside in the metropolitan areas of major cities. According to the 2000 US Census, the city with the largest percentage of Arab Americans is Dearborn, Michigan, a southwestern suburb of Detroit, at nearly 30%. The Detroit metropolitan area is home to almost 500,000, the largest concentration of those with an Arab heritage outside the Middle East.[23]

Rice and colleagues[19–21] conducted several studies in the Arab American youth population. Over 8 years, tobacco use data were collected from 2454 teens (14–18 years). The findings indicated that Arab American versus non–Arab American youth reported lower percentages of ever cigarette smoking (20% vs 39%), current cigarette smoking (7% vs 22%), and regular cigarette smoking (3% vs 15%). In contrast, Arab American versus non–Arab American youth reported significantly higher percentages of ever WPS (38% vs 21%) and current WPS (17% vs 11%). Seventy-seven percent of the students perceived WPS to be as harmful or more harmful than cigarette smoking.

Grade, race, and gender were significantly related to WP use. With regard to grade, students reported more experimental use of hookahs at higher grades (30% in the 9th grade vs 43% in the 12th grade), more social use of WPs in higher grades (9% in the 9th grade vs 21% in the 12th grade), and more addictive use of water pipes in higher grades (6% in the 9th grade vs 11% in the 12th grade). With regard to gender, boys (33%) reported higher experimental use than girls (20%), higher social use (13% vs 8%, respectively), and higher regular use (9% for boys and 3% for girls). Boys were 3 times more likely to engage in addictive use. Youth were more likely to be regular smokers if they had smoked the WP in the past 30 days (odds ratio [OR] = 1.6) and were more likely to be regular cigarette smokers if they also smoked WPs regularly (OR = 1.9). Age of first using a WP was predictive of regular WP use, but not of regular tobacco use.

The age of first smoking a whole cigarette was predictive of both regular WP and cigarette smoking. Contrary to expectations, these asymmetric results suggest that cigarette smoking rather than WP is a gateway behavior for Arab American youth. Logistic regression showed that youth were 11 times more likely to be currently smoking cigarettes if they currently smoked water pipes. Youth were also 11 times more likely to be current WP smokers if they currently smoked cigarettes. If one or more family members smoked WP in the home, youth were 6.3 times more likely to be current WP smokers. The effects of ethnicity were reduced as a result of the explanatory value of family smoking. The results of this study indicate that further research is necessary with youth to learn more about the potential for one form of tobacco use leading to another, given their close association and the relative health consequences of both. Other studies that have looked at adolescent WPS in the United States are those by Grekin and Ayna,[26] Primack and colleagues,[27] Smith-Simone and colleagues,[28] and Barnett and colleagues.[29] Studies of adult WP smokers include those by Jamil and colleagues.[30–32]

As the Arab and Arab American populations in this country have grown, so has the availability and use of WPs. Hookah bars or cafés have sprung up in urban and suburban areas and in cities and towns near large colleges and universities. Even a few of the states with strong smoke-free air laws have been unable to slow the growth of hookah bars and cafés. California, Illinois, New York, Texas, and Virginia currently have the largest number of these establishments; however, hookah bars and cafés have appeared in more than two-thirds of the states and there is growing concern about their health risk.[33] Based on US business listings and categorized Web listings, an estimated 200 to 300 of them currently operate in the United States, with more appearing every day.

## HEALTH PROBLEMS RELATED TO WPS

Recently, there have been several reviews on the negative effects of WPS on health outcomes.[10,34,35] In addition, findings from specific studies associate WPS with poor lung function,[36–38] malignant lung disease,[39] cancers of the mouth,[40] coronary heart disease,[41] perinatal risks,[42] and various other health problems. Cigarette smoking by adolescents is known to cause a number of health problems, including asthma, frequent respiratory infections, and impaired lung function,[43] but little is known about the effects of WP use with or without cigarette smoking on the respiratory function and health of adolescents.

One cannot assume that the lung and health consequences of these 2 types of smoking are the same, as they are performed in different ways with different doses and with different tobacco types. In addition, they produce different volumes of smoke, particulates, and nicotine.[44,45] One study[46] of hookah smokers found nicotine and cotinine increased up to 250% and 120%, respectively, after a typical 40-minute to 45-minute smoking session. WP use may increase exposure to carcinogens because smokers use a WP over a much longer period of time, often 40 to 45 minutes, rather than the 5 to 10 minutes it takes to smoke a cigarette. Because of the longer, more sustained period of inhalation and exposure, water pipe smokers may inhale as much smoke as consuming 100 or more cigarettes a single session.

## WPS INTERVENTION

Although there have been several trials that have tested interventions for cigarette smoking, Grimshaw and Stanton[47] reviewed 15 of them, showing moderate positive effects for successful cessation. No such trials were found for WPS.[48] Rice and colleagues[49] tested the effects of a prevention/cessation Project No Tobacco Use on cigarette and WPS in 380 Arab American and 236 non–Arab American ninth graders. Tenth-grade non–Arab American students (given the intervention as ninth graders) were 23% less likely to experiment (OR = 1.31, 95% confidence interval [CI]: 1.05, 1.64) or to have smoked cigarettes in the past 30 days (OR = 1.43 times, 95% CI: 1.03, 2.01) compared with Arab American youth. Arab American students reported greater experimentation with WPS than cigarettes (38% vs 22%), and more current (16% vs 6%) and regular (7% vs 3%) use of water pipes than cigarettes, respectively. The intervention (designed to focus on cigarette smoking) had little effect on WPS. These findings provide support for a school-based intervention revised to focus on prevention as well as cessation and to be culturally consistent. They also call for further research and intervention tailoring to address WPS in growing Arab and non–Arab American adolescent populations.

## SUMMARY

This article provides historical and current information on the growing threat of WPS around the world and in the United States. Not only is water pipe smoking prevalent in Middle Eastern culture, it has spread to all cultures. The evidence supports its greatest use among adolescents and young adults and a growing list of negative health problems are associated with its use. To date, no interventions have been designed and tested, but they are sorely needed. It continues to be the nurse's role to teach good health and no tobacco use to our clients, which means no WPS must be a part of every message.

## REFERENCES

1. WHO report on the Global Tobacco Epidemic 2011. World Health Organization; 2011. Available at: http://whqlibdoc.who.int/hq/2011/WHO.NMH_TFI_11.3_eng.pdf. Accessed September 9, 2011.
2. US Department of Health and Human Services. The health consequences of smoking: a report of the Surgeon General. Atlanta (GA): US Department of Health and Human Services, Centers for Disease Control and Prevention, National Center for Chronic Disease Prevention and Health Promotion, Office on Smoking and Health; 2004.
3. Behan DF, Eriksen MP, Lin Y. Economic effects of environmental tobacco smoke report (PDF–546.49 KB). Schaumburg (IL): Society of Actuaries; 2005.

4. Centers for Disease Control and Prevention. Smoking attributable mortality, morbidity, and economic costs (SAMMEC): adult SAMMEC and maternal and child health (MCH). SAMMEC software, 2002. Available at: http://www.cdc.gov/tobacco/sammec. Accessed September 10, 2011.

5. Centers for Disease Control and Prevention. Smoking-attributable mortality, years of potential life lost, and productivity losses—United States, 2000–2004. MMWR Morb Mortal Wkly Rep 2008;57(45):1226–8.

6. Shafey O, Musa D. Tobacco use: global perspective, Arab World, and Arab Americans. ACCESS Health 2010;1(1):37–43.

7. Hammal F, Mock J, Ward K, et al. A pleasure among friends: how narghile (waterpipe) smoking differs from cigarette smoking in Syria. Tob Control 2008;17:e3.

8. WHO study group on Tobacco Product Regualation (TobReg). Advisory Note. Waterpipe tobacco smoking: health effects, research needs, and recommended actions by regulators. Geneva: World Health Organization; 2005.

9. American Lung Association. An emerging deadly trend: waterpipe tobacco use. Washington, DC: American Lung Association; 2007.

10. Cobb C, Ward K, Maziak W, et al. Waterpipe tobacco smoking: an emerging health crisis in the United States. Am J Health Behav 2010;34(3):275–85.

11. Wolfram RM, Chehne F, Oguogho A, et al. Narghile (water pipe) smoking influences platelet function and (iso-)eicosanoids. Life Sci 2003;74:47–53.

12. Asotra K. The latest on Hookahs: what you don't know can kill you. Tobacco's Hottest Topics 2005;7(3):1–3. Available at: http://www.trdrp.org/Newsletters.asp. Accessed September 12, 2011.

13. Hadidi KA, Mohammed FI. Nicotine content in tobacco used in hubble-bubble smoking. Saudi Med J 2004;25:912–7.

14. Nakkashi RT, Khalil J, Afifi RA. The rise in narghile (shisha, hookah) waterpipe tobacco smoking: a qualitative study of perceptions of smokers and non smokers. BMC Pub Health 2011;11:315.

15. Al-Mulla AM, Helmy SA, Al-Lawati J, et al. Prevalence of tobacco use among students aged 13–15 years in Health Ministers' Council/Gulf Cooperation Council Member States, 2001–2004. J Sch Health 2008;78:337–43.

16. Akl EA, Gunukula SK, Aleem S, et al. The prevalence of waterpipe tobacco smoking among the general and specific populations: a systematic review. BMC Public Health 2011;11:244.

17. WHO REPORT on the global TOBACCO epidemic. mpower 2008. Available at: http://www.who.int/tobacco/mpower/mpower_report_full_2008.pdf. Accessed September 12, 2011.

18. Kandela P. Nargile smoking keeps Arabs in wonderland. Lancet 2000;356:1175.

19. Baker O, Rice V. Predictors of narghile (water-pipe) smoking in Yemeni American adolescents. J Transcult Nurs 2008;19:24–32.

20. Weglicki LS, Templin T, Hammad A, et al. Tobacco use patterns among high school students: do Arab American youth differ? Ethn Dis 2007;17(2 Suppl 3):22–4.

21. Rice VH, Templin T, Hammad A, et al. Collaboration study of tobacco use and its predictors in Arab and non Arab American 9th graders. Ethn Dis 2007; 17(2 Suppl 3):19–21.

22. Asfar T, Ward KD, Eissenberg T, et al. Comparison of patterns of use, beliefs, and attitudes related to waterpipe between beginning and established smokers. Nicotine Tob Res 2005;7(1):149–56.

23. Chaouachi K. Narghile (hookah): a socio-anthropological analysis. Culture, conviviality, history and tobaccology of a popular tobacco use mode. Paris: Université Paris X; 2000.

24. Maziak W, Eissenberg T, Rastam S, et al. Beliefs and attitudes related to narghile (waterpipe) smoking among university students in Syria. Ann Epidemiol 2004; 14(9):646–54.
25. The Arab American Institute. Available at: www.aaiusa.org/demographics. Accessed September 20, 2011.
26. Grekin ER, Ayna D. Argileh use among college students in the United States: an emerging trend. J Stud Alcohol Drugs 2008;69:472–5.
27. Primack BA, Walsh M, Bryce C, et al. Water-pipe tobacco smoking among middle and high school students in Arizona. Pediatrics 2009;123(2):e282–8.
28. Smith-Simone S, Maziak W, Ward KD, et al. Waterpipe tobacco smoking: knowledge, attitudes, beliefs, and behavior in two U.S. samples. Nicotine Tob Res 2008;10:393–8.
29. Barnett TE, Curbow BA, Weitz JR, et al. Water pipe tobacco smoking among middle and high school students. Am J Public Health 2009;99:2014. e19.
30. Jamil H, Rice VH, Hammad A, et al. Tobacco use of Arab American adults in Southeast Detroit. Iraqi Medical Journal 2006;52(1):56–61.
31. Jamil H, Templin T, Fakhouri M, et al. Comparison of personal characteristics, tobacco use, and health states in Chaldean, Arab American, and non-Middle Eastern White adults. J Immigr Minor Health 2008;10(2):245–8.
32. Jamil H, Elsouhag D, Hiller S, et al. Socio-demographic risk indicators of hookah smoking among White Americans: a pilot study. Nicotine Tob Res 2010;12: 525–9.
33. Noonan D. Exemptions for hookah bars in clean indoor air act legislation: a public health concern. Public Health Nurs 2010;27(1):49–53.
34. Akl EA, Gaddam S, Gunukula SK, et al. The effects of water pipe tobacco smoking on health outcomes: a systematic review. Int J Epidemiol 2010;39(3): 834–57.
35. Knishkowy B, Amitai Y. Water-pipe (narghile) smoking: an emerging health risk behavior. Pediatrics 2005;116:e113–9.
36. Kiter G, Ucan ES, Ceylan E, et al. Water-pipe smoking and pulmonary functions. Respir Med 2000;94:891–4.
37. Al-Fayez SF, Salleh M, Ardawi M, et al. Effects of sheesha and cigarette smoking on pulmonary function of Saudi males and females. Trop Geogr Med 1988;40: 115–23.
38. Raad D, Gaddam S, Schunemann HJ, et al. Effects of water pipe tobacco smoking on lung function: a systematic review and meta-analysis. Chest 2010; 139(4):764–74.
39. Hecht S. Tobacco carcinogens, their biomarkers and tobacco-induced cancer. Nat Rev Cancer 2003;3(10):733–44 (Nature Publishing Group).
40. El-Hakim IE, Uthman MA. Squamous cell carcinoma and keratoacanthoma of the lower lip associated with "Goza" and "Shisha" smoking. Int J Dermatol 1999;38: 108–10.
41. Jabbour S, El-Roueiheb Z, Sibai AM. Narghile (water-pipe) smoking and incident coronary heart disease: a case-control study. Ann Epidemiol 2003;13:570.
42. Nuwayhid I, Yamout B, Azar G, et al. Narghile (hubble-bubble) smoking, low birth weight, and other pregnancy outcomes. Am J Epidemiol 1998; 148:375–83.
43. Gold DR, Wang W, Wypil D, et al. Effects of cigarette smoking on lung function in adolescent boys and girls. N Engl J Med 1996;335:931–7.
44. Eissenberg T, Shihadeh A. Waterpipe tobacco and cigarette smoking: direct comparison of toxicant exposure. Am J Prev Med 2009;37(6):518–23.

45. Shihadeh A. Investigation of mainstream smoke aerosol of the argileh water pipe. Food Chem Toxicol 2003;41(1):143–52.
46. Shafagoj YA, Mohammed FI, Hadidi KA. Hubble-bubble (water pipe) smoking: levels of nicotine and cotinine in plasma, saliva and urine. Int J Clin Pharmacol Ther 2002;40(6):249–55.
47. Grimshaw GM, Stanton A. Tobacco cessation intervention for young people. Cochrane Database Syst Rev 2006;4:CD003289.
48. Maziak W, Ward KD, Eissenberg T. Interventions for waterpipe smoking cessation. Cochrane Database Syst Rev 2007;4:CD005549.
49. Rice VH, Weglicki L, Templin T, et al. Intervention effects on tobacco use in Arab and non–Arab American adolescents. Addict Behav 2009;25(3):507–16.

# Smokeless Tobacco: a Gender Analysis and Nursing Focus

Cameron White, PhD[a],*, John L. Oliffe, PhD, RN[b], Joan L. Bottorff, PhD, RN, FCAHS[c]

**KEYWORDS**

- Gender influences • Masculinity • Moist snuff
- Smokeless tobacco • Harm reduction

A mercurial feature of the tobacco landscape during the last quarter of the twentieth century through to the present has been the resurgence in the consumption of smokeless tobacco by men.[1–3] Historically, the main type of smokeless tobacco used in North America has been loose-leaf chewing tobacco, made from cut tobacco leaves. Chewing tobacco involved a great deal of spitting (expectorating) and was symbolically associated with the masculine virtues of settling the frontier, including a capacity for rough and physically demanding work. Chewing tobacco was so prominent that it was described as the "American Habit."[4]

The more recent resurgence in the consumption of smokeless tobacco has been marked by a shift from chewing tobacco and by a dramatic increase in the popularity of moist snuff, a granulated tobacco product that is also consumed orally. A small amount (a pinch) is placed between the lip and the teeth. The flavor and nicotine is released by sucking, rather than by chewing. Historically, moist snuff was only ever a marginal form of tobacco in North America. Its use was never widespread, and it was generally seen as dandified.[5] The contemporary popularity of moist snuff is therefore somewhat unprecedented, perhaps especially among men.

The rise of moist snuff can be understood as the result of 3 qualities or attributes. The first is that it is a spitless form of oral smokeless tobacco (ie, it requires no expectoration). The spitless aspect of moist snuff enables it to address social and moral concerns about spitting in public (historically associated with chewing tobacco) as well as concerns about the expulsion of smoke in public, which is widely viewed in

[a] School of Nursing, University of British Columbia, Vancouver Campus, 302-6190 Agronomy Road, Vancouver, BC, Canada V6T 1Z3
[b] School of Nursing, University of British Columbia, Vancouver Campus, T201 2211 Wesbrook Mall, Vancouver, BC, Canada V6T 2B5
[c] Institute for Healthy Living and Chronic Disease Prevention, University of British Columbia, Okanagan Campus, 3333 University Way, Kelowna, BC, Canada V1V 2B7
* Corresponding author.
*E-mail address:* Cameron.White@nursing.ubc.ca

Nurs Clin N Am 47 (2012) 149–157
doi:10.1016/j.cnur.2011.10.003
0029-6465/12/$ – see front matter © 2012 Elsevier Inc. All rights reserved.

contemporary society through a moral lens as inconsiderate and unsanitary as well as unhealthy.[6] The second aspect of the rise of moist snuff has been the way it has been promoted by the tobacco industry as less dangerous than cigarettes.[7] The third attribute of moist snuff has been its capacity to draw on the myths of masculinity associated with chewing tobacco. Thus, despite its historically marginalized position, moist snuff has come to be associated with genuine and authentic masculine ideals, perhaps especially within rural contexts.

In some respects, the qualities of moist snuff, its authentic masculinity on one hand and its cleanliness and health orientation on the other, seem to contradict each other. Yet, as this article argues, it is precisely the capacity of moist snuff to address these seemingly contradictory tendencies at the same time that have made it (1) extremely popular and (2) a significant health care challenge.

Many working in health care have responded to the rise of moist snuff by emphasizing that even if moist snuff is less dangerous than cigarette use, this in itself is no guarantee of safety. Given the massive global harms caused by cigarette smoking,[8] the legitimacy of espousing cigarette smoking as the benchmark against which to gauge the relative harm of smokeless tobacco, or anything else for that matter, is at best uncertain. Mejia and Ling[9] suggest that "Smokeless tobacco products are addictive, and their use has been linked to oral cancer, oropharyngeal cancer, heart disease, and pancreatic cancer." Others have argued that smokeless tobacco is a problem because its use encourages people to remain tobacco users who might otherwise have quit smoking in response to smoke-free environments.[10–12]

In light of the steady increase in the popularity of moist snuff, this article argues that the focus on the health concerns associated with moist snuff use can and should be supplemented with a gendered approach to the issue, whereby the prominence of men's consumption might be usefully addressed by men-centered nursing interventions.

## LOCATING SMOKELESS TOBACCO

In the nineteenth century, smokeless tobacco, in the form of chewing tobacco, was by far the most prevalent form of tobacco use in the United States. In 1880, for example, chewing tobacco represented more than 58% of all forms of tobacco consumed in America (followed by cigars at 25% and smoking tobacco at 13.5%).[13]

Chewing tobacco was used almost entirely by men. It was characterized by expectorating or spitting and was strongly associated with male locales, such as workplaces and sports fields (especially baseball fields), where there was easy access to spittoons and/or an abundance of open space.[14] The spitting that accompanied the practice was seen as inappropriate for, as well as around, women and was looked down on by the etiquette writers of the middle and upper classes.[15]

Chewing tobacco was differentiated according to the type of leaf used, the region it was grown, and method of production. The market was characterized by fierce competition and a high degree of brand loyalty. As one commentator put it, "Men may be argued with as to the steel they will put into their buildings, or the coal they will put into their furnaces, or the oil they will put into their lamps, or even the clothes they will wear, but argument cuts no figure with respect to the tobacco they chew."[16]

During the first half of the twentieth century, however, rates of consumption of chewing tobacco in the United States declined considerably. This decline was, in part, driven by the association between spitting and the spread of tuberculosis.[17,18] Slogans popularized by tuberculosis workers, such as "Spitting is dangerous, indecent and against the law" and "No spit, no consumption," took the attack against chewing to unprecedented heights.[15] The consumption of chewing tobacco was also affected by the rise of the cigarette.[19] As a result of these factors, between the 1920s and the 1970s, chewing tobacco became increasingly old fashioned and, at both a symbolic and practical level, was confined to "single, divorced, or widowed men living in the South or North Central area of the country who were employed only part-time or not at all."[20]

In the 1970s and 1980s, however, in the context of the great public health initiatives of the midtwentieth century, these smokeless tobacco trends started to reverse. Although rates of consumption of cigarettes gradually leveled off and subsequently declined, smokeless tobacco, including both chewing tobacco and moist snuff, started to reemerge as a viable, if not fashionable, form of tobacco use.

These increases in the use of smokeless tobacco, including both chewing tobacco and moist snuff, were most prominent in particular regions and amongst particular groups of men. It was prominent, for example, in the mountain states and in the southeast and southwest states of America, where up to 30% to 33% of young white men could be found using smokeless tobacco.[4,21] Smokeless tobacco use was also prominent amongst varsity football and baseball players. A 1989 National Collegiate Athletic Association (NCAA) survey of college athletes found a 40% increase in use from 1985 to 1989.[2,22] This same survey (1989) found that levels of smokeless tobacco use amongst NCAA baseball players had increased to an alarming 57%.[2,22]

Surveys by Philip Morris suggested that smokeless tobacco consumption could also be categorized by occupation. A 1981 study conducted by the Simmons Market Research Bureau, for example, found that smokeless tobacco use was common in occupations such as manufacturing, mining, construction, and agriculture, where smoking was prohibited and/or or the hands were used extensively in the provision of labor.[23] Another occupation in which smokeless tobacco consumption was particularly high was the military. A 1992 report found that between 25% and 33% of men younger than 24 years in the American Army, Navy, and Air Force had used smokeless tobacco products in the past year. This use was especially high among young men in the Marine Corps. Here, nearly half had used forms of smokeless tobacco within the last year.[20]

The reemergence of smokeless tobacco was driven by an increase in the consumption of both chewing tobacco and moist snuff. However, the most significant component of the increase in smokeless tobacco consumption was the popularity of moist snuff. Between 1978 and 1983, moist snuff consumption increased at nearly 4 times the rate of consumption of loose-leaf chewing tobacco. By 1983, moist snuff accounted for 62% of the entire smokeless tobacco market.[24] Mejia and Ling suggest that from 1982 to 2008, moist snuff remained the only growing segment of the smokeless tobacco market.[9,25] Understanding the increase in smokeless tobacco consumption amongst men in the late twentieth century (through to the present) therefore requires an analysis of the culture and meaning of moist snuff.

## MOIST SNUFF

The increase in the consumption of moist snuff has been almost entirely because of its use by men. The highest rates of growth have been among young men.[2] From 1970 to 1991, the prevalence of moist snuff use among all men aged 18 years and more increased from 1.5% to 3.3%; among men aged 18 to 24 years, however, it increased more than 8-fold, from 0.7% to 6.2%, making this age group the heaviest users of the product among those surveyed.[1,2] In addition to being young and of the male gender, most new users of most snuff have been white. As Connolly[2] illustrates in his work on oral snuff, the 1990 Youth Risk Behavior Survey found that 24% of all white male high school students had used moist snuff and other forms of smokeless tobacco at least once during the past month.

In addition to gender (men), race (white), and age (18–24 years), the increase in consumption of moist snuff can also be categorized in terms of geography. Its increase was most prominent in the traditional smokeless tobacco markets, in nonmetropolitan areas, and especially in the "mountain states, southeast and southwest U.S."[20] Rouse[4] also illustrates the rapid increase in moist snuff use in these regions. However, moist snuff also carried the use of smokeless tobacco into new areas. Moist snuff has been increasingly popular amongst consumers who, in the words of a market report conducted for Philip Morris, are "younger, better educated, less rural and [had] a higher income than traditional… users [of smokeless tobacco]."[20]

## MOIST SNUFF AND MASCULINITY

In the context of overrepresentation of men in the statistics concerning the increase in the consumption of smokeless tobacco in general, and moist snuff in particular, many commentators writing throughout the second half of the twentieth century have described the meanings and narratives invested in moist snuff use in terms of masculinity. A 1984 report for RJ Reynolds on "Why [Moist Snuff] is Growing in Popularity Among 18–24 Year Olds," for example, described its attractions in terms of it being "one of the few purely masculine activities left. [The] use of the product send[ing] a very clear signal about the masculinity of the user."[26]

This same report also emphasized the masculine ritualism associated with using the product as being very important and attractive to young men. It pointed, for example, to the importance of the "ring" imprint that snuff tins make in jean pockets as "a badge that identifies a user [as masculine] even if the product isn't in use."[26] A US Tobacco employee told a *New York Post* reporter that similarly "When a kid gets a new pair of jeans, he puts the snuff can in the back pocket and rubs it till the outline shows."[27]

The capacity of moist snuff to represent a sense of masculinity has mostly been seen to emanate from an association with rural life. One report suggested that moist snuff was "perceived as having rural roots."[26] A snuff user cited in a 1993 Philip Morris study entitled "A Qualitative Exploration of Snuff Category" described moist snuff as a "real Country Boy thing to do."[28] More specifically, moist snuff has been represented in terms of the Wild West. A report, commissioned by the British American Tobacco company in 1981, suggested that "A new and expanding youth franchise is developing within North America, to whom moist snuff has a genuine masculine, macho, cowboy sportsman country-and-western life style image which makes Marlboro in contrast seem like a phoney, [an] Urban-Cowboy-Adman's illusion."[19]

## SELLING POINTS OF MOIST SNUFF
### Cleanliness

Also central to the increase in popularity of moist snuff in recent times (in addition to its masculine appeal) has been the development of new forms of the product, such as Skoal Bandits, introduced by U.S. Tobacco in 1983, which have come in a convenient premoistened tea-bag–like pouch and are largely spitless.[29] These new products have been promoted by the tobacco industry on account of their capacity to avoid many of the concerns associated with masticating (chewing) and expectorating (spitting), which, in part, contributed to a decline in the social acceptability of chewing tobacco in the early part of the twentieth century.[15] In short, these new moist snuff products could be used discreetly, without being seen to do so (if desired).[19] As

Claude E. Teague Jr,[30] assistant chief in research and development at RJ Reynolds put it in 1971, "the juices can be swallowed and not spit out." Moreover, the small tea-bag–like packages were not "messy or unsightly to dispose of."[9,30] One report described the growth in the consumption of moist snuff in terms of its attractions for the "fastidious, hygiene-health orientated user who prefers discretion."[19] Another industry report suggested that "Smokeless tobacco may be overcoming its stigma as a rural, messy habit unsuitable for urban settings. This trend has been boosted by the increased popularity of moist snuff, which entails less expectoration and no visible 'cud' in the cheek. These characteristics allow for more convenient usage by white collar, urban individuals and may enhance the social acceptability of smokeless tobacco consumption."[23]

These new moist snuff products have also been promoted by the tobacco industry on account of the advantages they offer in relation to cigarettes.[20] The advantage of moist snuff in this respect has been that it has enabled tobacco consumers to negotiate the "problem" of smoke-free laws. It has therefore become particularly useful in the context of "dual use." Mejia and Ling[9] write in an analysis of more recent moist snuff products called snus, the Swedish term for oral moist snuff, that "Advertisements for Camel and Marlboro Snus tout it as a temporary way to deal with smoke-free policies in public places, bars, workplaces, and airplanes."

## Safety

A further advantage of smokeless tobacco in general, and moist snuff in particular, as argued by the tobacco industry, has been that it has been widely touted as a harm reduction measure because it is, statistically, less likely to cause cancer than cigarette smoking.[7] A 1981 report from the British American Tobacco, for example, highlighted that oral/moist snuff was the "most [commercially] interesting" form of smokeless tobacco and suggested, "It should stand up better to pressure and restrictions (on advertising and promotion, nicotine deliveries, smoking time and space, etc) than any type of smoking, and should get support from some medical and other authorities as an acceptable alternative to smoking."[19]

Representatives of the tobacco industry have also argued that smokeless tobacco, particularly moist snuff, can lead to a decrease in the number of cigarettes that smokers consume. In an article ostensibly about "smokeless tobacco," but which concentrated heavily on "the use of snus and moist smokeless tobacco products," Frost-Pineda and colleagues,[7] scientists employed by Altria (a "parent company" for Philip Morris, U.S. Smokeless Tobacco Company, and others), suggest that people who use smokeless tobacco and cigarettes (ie, dual users) are "more likely to reduce smoking intensity or to cease smoking cigarettes than exclusive smokers." Accordingly, "dual use… may result in reduction in smoking-related harm as smoking intensity is decreased and smoking cessation increases."

The debate about the relative harms of cigarette consumption versus the consumption of smokeless tobacco (particularly moist snuff) can be understood in terms of a longer history of projects initiated by the tobacco industry to represent itself as a responsible corporate citizen. These efforts have been designed, in the words of Benson,[31] to "capitalize on health risks to create an image of a caring industry that promotes lawful behavior, respects consumer autonomy, and works with and for the public health."

New moist snuff products have been promoted on account of their capacity to offer a cleaner and healthier version of smokeless tobacco designed to help consumers address concerns relating to other forms of smokeless tobacco as well as cigarettes. The proposed advantages of this new form of smokeless tobacco are that it is discrete, hygienic, convenient, and (relatively) healthy.

## MASCULINITY AND TECHNOLOGY

One of the most interesting aspects of moist snuff is the way in which its emphasis on virtues of cleanliness and hygiene and manners and etiquette seemed to contradict its claim to "genuine" white, rural, southern American masculinity. However, rather than viewing these attributes of moist snuff as contradictory, this article argues that they might best and most usefully be understood as complimenting each other. In other words, it was precisely the technical advances associated with moist snuff that allowed its genuine southern, rural, masculine appeal to cross over to a wider, younger, better-educated, urban/metropolitan, white collar, middle-class audience. Mejia and Ling write, "Although tobacco users participating in [market] research associated moist snuff with outdoor men, with rugged, individualistic people who worked in places where they could not smoke, and with farm or rural backgrounds, they did not perceive moist snuff to be as ''low class'' as other chewing tobacco."[9]

In the context of its crossover appeal, the increase in moist snuff can be seen to have done 2 things. It has reinvigorated the appeal of smokeless tobacco amongst a particular culture of rural white American masculinity. At the same time, however, moist snuff can also be seen to have had a more general effect in that it has reinvigorated the appeal of rural white American masculinity and made it more attractive, desirable, and accessible to a wider constituency. This emphasis on the social and gendered significance of moist snuff draws on the work of Latour[32] who not only illustrates the extent to which technologies such as, in this case, new forms of smokeless tobacco (ie, moist snuff) reflect the social order, as if "the 'reflected' society existed somewhere else," but also argues that these "technologies" (ie, moist snuff) are "in large part the stuff out of which socialness is made." This article argues that health care interventions, to be effective, need to consider the social significance of moist snuff as well as its capacity to affect the health of users.

## IMPLICATIONS FOR NURSES AND OTHER HEALTH CARE PROVIDERS

The use of moist snuff has encouraged the development and evaluation of interventions to support cessation. In a recent review of randomized trials on behavioral or pharmacologic interventions to help users of smokeless tobacco to quit, the investigators concluded that nicotine replacement therapy (including gum and patches) does not help with long-term cessation.[33] Behavioral interventions such as social support via regular telephone counseling as well as oral examinations and feedback about smokeless tobacco–induced mucosal changes were suggested. Further research is needed to identify effective approaches for the unique groups of smokeless tobacco users. The social and gendered meanings of smokeless tobacco described in this article provide direction for tailored interventions and health promotion efforts.

Nurses and other health care providers have tended to respond to the popularity of smokeless tobacco by highlighting the health dangers posed by its use. For example, an emphasis on the relationship between smokeless tobacco and cancer[9] has been used to catalyze strong objections to a harm reduction approach. In this respect, the authors suggest that smokeless tobacco be addressed in ways that are delinked from both harm reduction and cigarette smoking. The risks of smokeless tobacco need to be compartmentalized and highlighted as unique considerations worthy of focused interventions. The authors' recommendation for a delinked approach is supported by Glantz and Ling who assert that smokeless tobacco encourages people to remain tobacco users who might otherwise have quit smoking in response to smoke-free environments.[10] Tomar and colleagues[11] argue, similarly, that there is little evidence that smokeless tobacco is effective in the promotion of harm reduction, and Hatsukami and colleagues[12] write, "promulgating noncombusted oral tobacco products as a safer alternative to smoking or as a substitute for smoking may engender more rather than less harm."

In arguing for a delinked approach, several key considerations emerge regarding how we might best support men to reduce or cease using smokeless tobacco in gender-sensitive ways. In this regard, previous work on tobacco reduction and smoking cessation provides some important clues. For example, a semiotic analysis of professionally produced smoking cessation image–based campaigns by Johnson and colleagues[34] revealed scare tactics as having little impact, although more subtle messaging about not fulfilling particular masculine roles (ie, breadwinner and fathering) as a byproduct of tobacco-induced illness has been shown to influence tobacco reduction among new dads who smoked. In this regard, public health and health promotion nurses might thoughtfully consider the usage of similar subtle campaigns to message subgroups of men, including college men in attempting to dislocate connections between masculine ideals and smokeless tobacco.

The testimonials of men who are attempting to quit, or have recently quit, smokeless tobacco might also provide an effective approach to men-centered interventions. The authors base this recommendation, in part, on a recent study from which a booklet privileging the testimonials of new dads who smoke but want to reduce or quit were used to provide empathy and strategies for reducing smoking amid acknowledging the challenges for making such changes.[35] This approach can bypass the exclusive emphasis on the health dangers posed by smokeless tobacco, an argument whose efficacy is easily limited by the tobacco industry's ability to transform the debate into a tit-for-tat, "yes it is (dangerous)," "no it is not" exchange.[10,36] In addition, the testimonials of other men can be used to situate the question of consumption of smokeless tobacco as ultimately a matter of opinion in ways that appeal to masculine ideals around strength and self-discipline in making the decision to reduce or quit.

Nurses can also perform, as well as foster, interprofessional approaches (ie, dentists, dental hygienists) to raise awareness of the availability of oral cancer screening. For example, targeted screening might be aimed at a high-risk subpopulation, including college men, as a means to highlighting potential problems early on as well as raising awareness of the connections between smokeless tobacco and health-related risks.

As this article demonstrates, approaches to intervening around smokeless tobacco will be well served by focusing on the masculinities with which it is intricately associ-ated. The focus on masculinity, however, is relational, and, as Connell[37] reminds, first and foremost masculinity is a way of ordering social relations, both between men and women as well as between men. In this respect, although smokeless tobacco resides predominately as a men's issue, there is great potential for the practices to be restrained or embodied by "significant others." Likewise, there may also be some credence in messaging men through the women and men in their lives to inform smokeless tobacco users about the unattractive nature of that practice in promoting cessation. Researchers examining the impact of social support provided by female partners (n = 328) of male participants in a smokeless tobacco cessation program have reported that positive support and encouragement from partners can encourage long-term cessation.[38]

## SUMMARY

Concerns have been raised about the increasing consumption of smokeless tobacco, particularly in the form of moist snuff, among specific subgroups of men. These trends are a response to promotion of moist snuff by the tobacco industry as a healthier, more convenient, smoke-free alternative to cigarettes and as an especially masculine form of tobacco consumption. The health risks of smokeless tobacco and the social and gendered meanings of smokeless tobacco provide direction for health promotion efforts. Men-centered approaches to raising awareness about the connections between smokeless tobacco and oral cancer and the availability of oral cancer screening are 2 key nursing practice considerations.

## REFERENCES

1. Giovino GA, Schooley MW, Zhu B, et al. Surveillance for selected tobacco-use behaviors: United States, 1900-1994. MMWR CDC Surveill Summ 1994; 43(SS3):1–43.
2. Connolly GN. The marketing of nicotine addiction by one oral snuff manufacturer. Tob Control 1995;4(1):73–9.
3. Centers for Disease Control. Tobacco use among high school students–United States, 1990. MMWR Morb Mortal Wkly Rep 1991;40(36):617–9.
4. Rouse BA. Epidemiology of smokeless tobacco use: a national study. NCI Monogr 1989;8:29–33.
5. Burns E. The smoke of the gods: a social history of tobacco. Philadelphia: Temple University Press; 2007.
6. Poland BD. The 'considerate' smoker in public space: the micro-politics and political economy of 'doing the right thing'. Health Place 2000;6(1):1–14.
7. Frost-Pineda K, Appleton S, Fisher M, et al. Does dual use jeopardize the potential role of smokeless tobacco in harm reduction? Nicotine Tob Res 2010;12(11): 1055–67.
8. Proctor RN. Tobacco and the global lung cancer epidemic. Nat Rev Cancer 2001; 1(1):82–6.
9. Mejia AB, Ling PM. Tobacco industry consumer research on smokeless tobacco users and product development. Am J Public Health 2010;100(1):78–87.
10. Glantz SA, Ling PM. Misleading conclusions from Altria researchers about population health effects of dual use. Nicotine Tob Res 2011;13(4):296.
11. Tomar SL, Fox BJ, Severson HH. Is smokeless tobacco use an appropriate public health strategy for reducing societal harm from cigarette smoking? Int J Environ Res Public Health 2009;6(1):10–24.
12. Hatsukami DK, Ebbert JO, Feuer RM, et al. Changing smokeless tobacco products—new tobacco-delivery systems. Am J Prev Med 2007;33(6):S368–78.
13. Milmore BK, Conover AG. Tobacco consumption in the United States, 1880–1955. In: Haenszel W, Shimkin MB, Miller HP, editors. Tobacco smoking patterns in the United States. Washington, DC: U.S. Government Printing Office; 1956. p. 107–11.
14. Morris P. Personally, I have nothing against smoking: the lethal alliance between baseball and the cigarette. NINE: A Journal of Baseball History and Culture 2009; 18(1):37–62.
15. Tomes N. The gospel of germs: men, women, and the microbe in American life. Boston: Harvard University Press; 1999.
16. Supreme Court of the United States. The United States of America against the American Tobacco Company and others. In the supreme court of the United States, 316. 1908. Available at: http://legacy.library.ucsf.edu/tid/qzj64a00. Accessed July 29, 2011.
17. Chapman S. Great expectorations! The decline of public spitting: lessons for passive smoking? BMJ 1995;311(7021):1685–6.

18. Goodman J. Tobacco in history: the cultures of dependence. New York: Routledge; 1993.
19. Pearson. Smokeless tobacco. 1981; Bates Number 300040460–300040494. Available at: http://legacy.library.ucsf.edu/tid/yku08a99. Accessed July 27, 2011.
20. Lembo L. Smokeless tobacco industry analysis. 1993; Bates Number 2046710489/0509. Available at: http://tobaccodocuments.org/pm/2046710489-0509; http://legacy.library.ucsf.edu/tid/vpt92e00. Accessed July 25, 2011.
21. National Cancer Institute. Smokeless tobacco or health: an international perspective. Smoking and tobacco control monograph no. 2. Washington: National Institute of Health; 1992.
22. Anderson WA, Albrecht RR, McKeag DB. Second replication of the National Study of the substance use and abuse habits of college student-athletes. East Lansing (MI): Michigan State University; 1993.
23. Long HP, Plskor SK. Smokeless tobacco. 1984; Bates Number 2040272649/2654. Available at: http://tobaccodocuments.org/pm/2040272649-2654.html; http://legacy.library.ucsf.edu/tid/gfd05e00. Accessed July 25, 2011.
24. Morris P. Smokeless tobacco. 1984; Bates Number: 2040272649/2654. Available at: http://legacy.library.ucsf.edu/tid/gfd05e00. Accessed July 25, 2011.
25. Reynolds RJ. 1983-1987 plan. 1982; Bates Number 502480001/0220. Available at: http://tobaccodocuments.org/rjr/500402517-2570.html. Accessed July 19, 2011.
26. Bellis JV. RJR younger adult users of moist snuff. 1984. Available at: http://legacy.library.ucsf.edu/tid/uhd95d00. Accessed July 19, 2011.
27. Heald H. Carlis cole, plaintiffs, v the Tobacco Institute, Inc, defendants. Plaintiff original complaint. 1997. Available at: http://legacy.library.ucsf.edu/tid/hfk43c00. Accessed July 23, 2011.
28. Marketing perceptions. A qualitative exploration of snuff category. 1993; Bates Number 2045722574/2590. Available at: http://legacy.library.ucsf.edu/tid/afb07e00. Accessed July 23, 2011.
29. Morris P. Smokeless tobacco. Inter-office correspondence. 1984. Available at: http://legacy.library.ucsf.edu/tid/gfd05e00. Accessed July 21, 2011.
30. Teague C. Research planning memorandum on modified chewing tobacco-like products. 1971; Bates Number 502987378/7382. Available at: http://legacy.library.ucsf.edu/tid/aqd53d00. Accessed July 21, 2011.
31. Benson P. Safe cigarettes. Dialect Anthropol 2010;34:49–56.
32. Latour B. When things strike back: a possible contribution of 'science studies' to the social sciences. Br J Sociol 2000;51(1):107–23.
33. Ebbert J, Montori VM, Erwin PJ, et al. Interventions for smokeless tobacco use cessation. Cochrane Database Syst Rev 2011;2:CD004306.
34. Johnson JL, Oliffe JL, Kelly MT, et al. The readings of smoking fathers: a reception analysis of tobacco cessation images. Health Commun 2009;24(6):532–47.
35. Oliffe JL, Bottorff JL, Sarbit G. Mobilizing masculinity to support fathers who want to be smoke free: CIHR Institute of Gender and Health knowledge translation casebook. Canadian Institute for Health Research: Ottawa; 2011.
36. Rodu B. Dual use. Nicotine Tob Res 2011;13(3):221.
37. Connell R, Messerschmidt J. Hegemonic masculinity—rethinking the concept. Gend Soc 2005;19(6):829–59.
38. Danaher BG, Lichtenstein E, Andrews JA, et al. Women helping chewers: effects of partner support on 12-month tobacco abstinence in a smokeless tobacco cessation trial. Nicotine Tob Res 2009;11(3):332–5.

# E-Cigarettes: Promise or Peril?

Carol A. Riker, MSN, RN[a],*, Kiyoung Lee, ScD, MPH[b,c],
Audrey Darville, APRN, CTTS[b,d], Ellen J. Hahn, PhD, RN[a]

KEYWORDS

- Tobacco • Policy • Smoking cessation • Smoke-free
- Harm reduction • Addiction

This article provides an overview of the history, production, and marketing of e-cigarettes, the contents of e-cigarettes and vapor, how they are used, public health concerns, and implications for nursing practice, research, and policy development. Current information was gathered by searching the professional literature and monitoring relevant websites and listservs. This article does not provide a comprehensive, systematic review of the pharmacokinetics and pharmacodynamics of e-cigarette use.

## MECHANISM OF ACTION

E-cigarettes are battery-operated devices that contain cartridges generally filled with nicotine, flavor and other chemicals.[1,2] Puffing activates a battery-operated heating element in the atomizer and the solution in the cartridge is vaporized and inhaled (**Fig. 1**).[3] Because e-cigarettes do not burn tobacco, they do not emit smoke. Rather, the user inhales and exhales a vapor, also called a plume, fog, or aerosol.[4–6] Most e-cigarettes are designed to look like traditional cigarettes and simulate the visual, sensory, and behavioral aspects of smoking traditional cigarettes.[7,8] However, some e-cigarettes look like everyday items such as pens and USB memory sticks that may go unnoticed.[9] E-cigarette cartridges can be refilled using drops of solution sold in bottles, some of which contain more than 500 mg of nicotine, approximately 10

Funding: Funding was provided by the Kentucky Department for Public Health and the Foundation for a Healthy Kentucky. This work was partially supported by the National Research Foundation of Korea Grant funded by the Korean Government (NRF-2011-013-D00068).
Disclosures: The authors have nothing to disclose.
[a] Tobacco Policy Research Program, Kentucky Center for Smoke-free Policy, University of Kentucky College of Nursing, 751 Rose Street, Lexington, KY 40536-0232, USA
[b] Tobacco Policy Research Program, University of Kentucky College of Nursing, 751 Rose Street, Lexington, KY 40536-0232, USA
[c] Graduate School of Public Health, Seoul National University, 1 Gwanak-ro, Gwanak-gu, Seoul 115-742, Korea
[d] UKHealthCare, 800 Rose Street, Lexington, KY 40536, USA
* Corresponding author.
E-mail address: riker@email.uky.edu

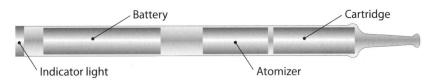

Fig. 1. E-cigarette components. (*Courtesy of* University of Kentucky. Copyright © 2011, University of Kentucky.)

times the lethal dose.[3] Pauly and colleagues[10] described the stated or implied intent of e-cigarettes as reducing toxins in the mainstream and secondhand smoke and helping smokers quit.

### History of the Product, FDA Regulation, Current Marketing, and Profits

E-cigarettes were introduced into European markets in 2006 and American markets in 2007.[11] Because of the rapid increase in use and uncertainty about the chemical contents and their safety, the FDA blocked new shipments in 2008 under its authority to regulate drugs, drug delivery devices, or drug/device combinations under the Food, Drug, and Cosmetic Act (FDCA).[12] In July 2009, the FDA released laboratory analyses of a few e-cigarette samples and issued a public warning that e-cigarettes may contain carcinogens and toxic chemicals, as well as nicotine (which is highly addictive). In this warning, the FDA expressed concern about safety and marketing, including marketing to youth over the Internet and at mall kiosks.[1] In September 2010, the FDA sent warning letters to five e-cigarette manufacturers[13] and wrote to the Electronic Cigarette Association inviting firms to work with the agency toward lawful marketing of e-cigarettes in the United States.[9]

In 2009, the FDA blocked import of a shipment from Sottera, an importer and distributor, claiming authority under the FDCA.[14] Sottera, Inc. challenged the authority of the FDA to prevent import of its e-cigarettes, saying they serve the same purpose as cigarettes, and therefore should be regulated under the Tobacco Act.[14] The District Court agreed and an appeal was filed. The US Court of Appeals for the Washington, DC Circuit decided in December 2010 that e-cigarettes can be regulated as "tobacco products" under the Family Smoking Prevention and Tobacco Control Act of 2009 and that they are not drugs/devices unless therapeutic claims are made. In a letter to stakeholders, the FDA announced the court decision and its intent to regulate e-cigarettes as tobacco products and to consider issuing a "guidance" and/or regulation on "therapeutic" claims.[15] As of September 2011, the FDA was in the initial process of drafting a regulation; they will invite public comment and analyze the comments before a final regulation is issued.[12] When this regulation will be implemented or how broad it will be were unknown as of September 2011.

Meanwhile, those who support and manufacture alternative smoking products have become increasingly interested in the potential to enlarge their customer base and increase profits.[2] At least three major US organizations promote and advocate for e-cigarettes and other alternatives to smoking, including the Electronic Cigarette Association, the Consumer Advocates for Smoke-Free Alternatives Association (CASAA), and Vapers International, Inc.[11] In 2010, the National Vapers Club estimated that at least 1 million people in the United States used e-cigarettes and that the number of e-cigarette companies had risen to approximately 300.[16] In January 2009, Ruyan Group, Ltd. reported worldwide revenues of approximately $54 million and Vapor Corp reported $7.95 million in US sales.[11]

Internet marketing has proliferated through Web sites, social networking sites such as Facebook, YouTube promotional videos, advertising on search engines, and

Internet forums that host sessions on how to use e-cigarettes.[11] Other marketing outlets include mall kiosks, tobacco retail stores, and contracts with gasoline station distributors. Users can become distributors and recruit customers for profit.[4] In minutes, one can become a salesperson with access to posters, pamphlets, and business cards, and a Web forum exists for sharing online marketing strategies.[4] Marketing includes high-tech perks, such as a charging outlet that has a USB port so that e-cigarettes can be recharged on a computer. Some e-cigarettes even have global positioning systems that help the user network with other e-cigarette users nearby to promote social use of the product.[17] E-cigarette marketing patterns are similar to tobacco marketing strategies in that they have entered the world of Hollywood, with appearances in popular movies, television talk shows, and even in the gift bags given the nominees at the 2011 Academy Awards.[18]

The FDA and other health agencies remain concerned about how e-cigarettes are marketed to the public and the possibility that they may promote nicotine addiction, delay or derail serious quit attempts, and encourage youth tobacco use. Marketing that portrays e-cigarettes as products that can be used where smoking is prohibited has the potential to cause confusion in the implementation and enforcement of smoke-free policies. Use of e-cigarettes continues to model smoking as an adult norm and may increase the risk of nicotine addiction among youth and young adults.[19] Flavored e-cigarettes marketed as "green" and "healthy" may serve as a new starter product for nonusers. Users who look to e-cigarettes as a cessation aid may not achieve success and may become dual users (using e-cigarettes where smoking is prohibited and continuing their use of traditional cigarettes or other tobacco products where allowed). Some suggest that e-cigarettes would only be of public health benefit if they help smokers completely quit smoking traditional cigarettes.[7]

## WHAT DO E-CIGARETTES AND THE VAPOR CONTAIN?

Currently more than 300 brands of e-cigarettes are available, although testing has been conducted on only a few brands, primarily by the FDA and Health New Zealand (e-cigarettes and funding were supplied under a contract with Ruyan [Holdings] Ltd Hong Kong, now doing business as Dragonite International Limited). A Greek study mentioned by several authors was not accessible. Research completed by the Korean National Evidence-based Healthcare Collaborating Agency was provided by coauthor Lee.[20] Clearly, a dearth of scientific evidence exists on the safety or efficacy of e-cigarettes.

### Nicotine

Nicotine is a unique chemical found in tobacco products. Nicotine stimulates mammals at low concentrations and is the main chemical responsible for the dependence-forming properties of tobacco smoking and some of the cardiovascular effects.[21] It is highly toxic and can be purchased as a pesticide in some parts of the world. Because vapor from e-cigarettes contains nicotine, exposure to the vapor can be harmful to smokers and bystanders. The presence of nicotine in cartridges and vapor from e-cigarettes can be hazardous. Refills may contain high levels of nicotine[22] and pose dangers to users and nonusers from leaky cartridges, fluid remaining in spent cartridges, and dermal exposure to nicotine while loading refills.[23] Additionally, nicotine from the vapor or from cartridge fluid sticks to surfaces for weeks or months, reacting over time with nitrous acid in the air to form carcinogens, exposing bystanders via inhalation, ingestion, or dermal exposure.[19,24]

Nicotine has been found in e-cigarette cartridges, even when the product label does not include nicotine.[25,26] The FDA's analysis showed that cartridges labeled "high" had the highest nicotine concentration, as shown in **Fig. 2**.[25] However, the nicotine content in similarly labeled cartridges varied. For example, a product labeled "low nicotine" contained more nicotine than one labeled "medium." Additionally, many products labeled as having no nicotine actually contained nicotine; the FDA report detected nicotine in four of five of these cartridges.[25] Hadwiger and colleagues[26] reported that all five e-cigarette cartridges labeled as containing no nicotine actually contained the drug. Furthermore, products may emit different amounts of nicotine with each puff (26.8–43.2 μg of nicotine per 100-mL puff).[25] A nicotine concentration of 0.35 μg per 100-mL puff was measured in cartridges labeled as containing no nicotine.

### *Propylene Glycol*

Propylene glycol, a chemical found in theater "smoke," cosmetics, and foods, is typically used to make the "vapor" emitted from e-cigarettes.[2] However, a major industrial company recommends that inhalation exposure to mists of propylene glycol be avoided.[27] Varughese and colleagues[28] studied 101 employees at 19 sites using glycol or mineral oil theatrical fogs, measured personal fog exposure, and found that the fogs have the potential to generate acute and chronic respiratory effects. They also reported reduced lung function with increased proximity to the fog and with cumulative exposure.[28] Reduction and elimination of exposure to these theatrical fogs were recommended. The American Chemistry Council (ACC) expressed concern about transient eye pain, conjunctivitis, and tearing from a single contact with theater fog containing propylene glycol.[29] The ACC recommended that those exposed to propylene glycol wear eye protection and avoid use of contact lenses.[29] The tobacco and pharmaceutical industries have conducted studies on the safety of inhaling aerosolized propylene glycol, but no human studies have been published.[30,31]

Westenberger[25] detected diethylene glycol, an impurity of propylene glycol, in one e-cigarette cartridge. Like propylene glycol, diethylene glycol is colorless and

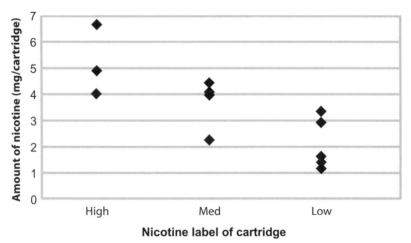

**Fig. 2.** Nicotine content of e-cigarettes correlated with levels indicated on label. (*Data from* Westenberger BJ. Evaluation of e-cigarettes. U.S. Food and Drug Association, 2009. Available at: http://www.fda.gov/downloads/Drugs/ScienceResearch/UCM173250.pdf. Accessed August 22, 2011.)

odorless. However, diethylene glycol is highly toxic and has resulted in poisoning epidemics since the early 20th century.[32] Because of its adverse effects on humans, diethylene glycol is not allowed in food and drugs.

## Other Contents

Very few studies have been conducted on the chemical contents of e-cigarettes and vapor, and these studies tested a limited number of products. Therefore, the chemicals listed in **Table 1** do not represent all chemicals contained in e-cigarettes, and concentrations of the chemicals in the cartridges and vapor are not presented. Several other toxic chemicals have been found in e-cigarette cartridges. Hadwiger and colleagues[26] reported that some e-cigarettes also deliver drugs for weight loss or erectile dysfunction. One cartridge labeled to contain Cialis did not, but contained amino-tadalafil. Another cartridge containing rimonabant was correctly marked. This chemical may have been added to promote weight control, but it is not approved for use in the United States.

Tobacco-specific nitrosamines, including N-nitrosonornicotine, N-nitrosoanabasine, N-nitrosoanatabine, 4-(methylnitrosamino)-1-(3-pyridyl)-1-butanone have been detected in e-cigarette cartridges.[25,33] Nitrosamines are known carcinogens. Anabasine and myosmine are alkaloids found in tobacco and are chemically similar to nicotine. β-Nicotyrine is an alkaloid derived from the dehydrogenation of nicotine. Anabasine, myosmine, and β-nicotyrine were detected in the cartridges, and β-nicotyrine was measured in the vapor. In addition, several volatile organic compounds were detected in the cartridges, the vapor, or both. Among the volatile compounds, formaldehyde, a known carcinogen, was detected in both the cartridge and the vapor.[20,33] Considering the potential health effects from the known constituents, the inhaled compounds and the vapor from e-cigarettes are of public health concern.

Currently, no standard method exists to test e-cigarette vapor. The FDA analysis applied a trapping device consisting of a 150-mL gas-washing bottle with a sparger.[25] Air was drawn in using a 100-cm$^3$ hand pump. The Health New Zealand experiment applied a disposable plastic syringe connected to the e-cigarette with a short plastic tubing.[33] A smoker's puff was simulated by a moderately rapid pull on the syringe plunger. Because the air drawing speed and puff volume may influence the amount of mist and concentration of solvents, standardization of the experimental method to test the vapor is needed. Extensive testing of cartridges and refills is necessary to standardize the product and test for safety.[3,7]

## HOW ARE E-CIGARETTES USED AND ARE THEY EFFECTIVE FOR SMOKING CESSATION?

At least three online surveys related to e-cigarette use have been conducted. Etter[34] surveyed 81 ever-users who mainly used e-cigarettes to quit smoking and found them helpful. However, the sample was self-selected and could have oversampled satisfied, long-term, or heavy users. Participants expressed worry about the potential toxicity of the products. The median duration of use was similar to the median duration of abstinence in former smokers (100 days). Siegel and colleagues[35] surveyed 222 respondents in a nonconvenience sample of the first 5000 purchasers from a particular distributor. The authors reported a 31% 6-month smoking abstinence rate. Limitations noted by the authors were that abstinence was self-reported (no biochemical verification), no information was provided on nonresponders (despite a very low participation rate), and users of only one brand were surveyed. Etter and Bullen[36] surveyed 3587 participants recruited by an online survey in English and French posted on a smoking cessation Web site. Researchers contacted e-cigarette Web sites and forums

**Table 1**
**Chemicals found in e-cigarette cartridges and vapor**

| Chemical | Characteristics | Detection Media | Reference (Funding Source) |
|---|---|---|---|
| Amino-tadalafil | Drug analog of the commercially approved Cialis (tadalafil) | Cartridge for e-cigarette labeled to contain Cialis | Hadwiger et al,[26] 2010 (FDA) |
| Rimonabant | Drug that was, at one time, approved for weight loss in Europe, but not in the United States (approval has since been retracted) | Cartridge for e-cigarette labeled to contain rimonabant | Hadwiger et al,[26] 2010 (FDA) |
| N-nitrosonornicotine N-nitrosoanabasine N-nitrosoanatabine 4-(methyl-nitrosamino)-1-(3-pyridyl)-1-butanone | Tobacco-specific nitrosamines are strong carcinogens present in cigarette smoke | E-cigarette cartridge | Westenberger,[25] 2009 (FDA) Laugesen[33] (Health New Zealand)[a] |
| Anabasine | Pyridine alkaloid found in the tree tobacco (Nicotiana glauca) plant, a close relative of the common tobacco plant (Nicotiana tabacum) | E-cigarette cartridge | Westenberger,[25] 2009 (FDA) |
| Myosmine | Alkaloid found in tobacco | E-cigarette cartridge | Westenberger,[25] 2009 (FDA) |
| β-nicotyrine | Alkaloid derived from the dehydrogenation of nicotine | Cartridge and vapor | Westenberger,[25] 2009 (FDA) |
| Diethylene glycol | An ingredient used in antifreeze Toxic to humans | E-cigarette cartridge | Westenberger,[25] 2009 (FDA) |
| Ethyl alcohol Acetaldehyde | Many volatile organic compounds can cause health effects | E-cigarette cartridge and vapor | Laugesen[33] (Health New Zealand)[a] |
| Acetone Cresol Xylene Styrene | Many volatile organic compounds can cause health effects | Vapor | Laugesen[33] (Health New Zealand)[a] |
| Formaldehyde | Carcinogen | E-cigarette cartridge Vapor | National Evidence-based Healthcare Collaborating Agency (Korean government) Laugesen[33] (Health New Zealand)[a] |

*Abbreviation:* USFDA, US Food and Drug Administration.
[a] Industry-supported.
*Data from* Refs.[20,25,26,33]

requesting that they publish the link to the survey. Most participants reported using e-cigarettes to quit smoking or avoid relapse (77%) or deal with withdrawal or cravings (67%). Users also shared that e-cigarettes were less expensive than smoking (57%), and they perceived them to be less toxic than tobacco (84%). Limitations included selection bias and a potential for oversampling satisfied or heavy/long-term users.

McQueen and colleagues[6] interviewed a very small convenience sample of participants (N = 15) attending the MidWest Vapefest in St. Louis and other meetings of the MidWest Vapers Group. Participants were interviewed in small groups or individually. Some recurring themes were that (1) friends, advertisements, and Internet sites were common ways of learning about e-cigarettes; (2) learning to use e-cigarettes is complex; (3) perceived benefits of e-cigarette use included decreased cost, close approximation to the traditional smoking experience, weight control, fewer negative health effects, and increased ability to be physically active; (4) participants reported reduced nicotine tolerance and dependence; and (5) participants were interested in reading about and participating in advocacy and research. A unique language that mixed technical, pseudo-technical and popular jargon was observed. The authors noted that future research is urgently needed to compare e-cigarettes with both nicotine replacement products and traditional cigarettes.[6] Contrary to findings in Benowitz's[21] review, McQueen and colleagues[6] claim that nicotine contributes to few of the long-terms health problems of smoking, as does Rodu,[8] in his article entitled "The Scientific Foundation for Tobacco Harm Reduction."

Capponetto and colleagues[37] presented a case study of two smokers treated at a smoking cessation clinic who were clinically depressed and had a history of relapse. At a follow-up visit, both reported using e-cigarettes to quit smoking on their own (quit status measured objectively). Both clients had abstained from smoking traditional cigarettes for at least 6 months at the time of the report.

Other studies describe the pharmacokinetics and pharmacodynamics of e-cigarettes. Bullen and colleagues[38] randomized 40 adult dependent smokers to four study groups: e-cigarettes with 16 mg of nicotine, e-cigarettes with 0 mg of nicotine, nicotine inhaler, or usual brand of cigarette. No difference was seen in the desire to smoke between the 16-mg e-cigarette and nicotine inhaler groups, but subjects reported less mouth and throat irritation with the e-cigarette. The pharmacokinetic profile with the 16-mg e-cigarette was similar to that with the nicotine inhaler. Vansickel and colleagues[39] studied 32 smokers assigned to four independent Latin-square ordered conditions differing according to product (own brand traditional cigarette, e-cigarette with 18-mg of nicotine, e-cigarette with 16 mg of nicotine, or an unlit cigarette). Neither e-cigarette exposed users to measurable nicotine or carbon monoxide, and neither increased heart rate. E-cigarettes produced some reduction in withdrawal symptoms, although less than their own brand.

Trtchounian and colleagues[40] used a smoking machine to conclude that taking stronger puffs was needed to smoke e-cigarettes than regular cigarettes and that the puff strength needed to be increased over the course of using the e-cigarette. Characteristics such as puff strength and aerosol density varied widely within and between e-cigarette brands.

## THE ROLE OF E-CIGARETTES IN THE "HARM REDUCTION" DEBATE

Well-formulated evidence-based clinical practice guidelines exist for tobacco dependence treatment, but, at best, the abstinence rates for people using these treatments remain low.[41,42] Tobacco use is a chronic, relapsing disease involving addiction to nicotine.[43] One way to treat tobacco addiction is to suggest a variety of approved, effective cessation medications, including nicotine delivery devices. However, therapeutic nicotine replacement products are slower and less efficient at delivering nicotine, which makes their use less satisfying to most users than the tobacco product. Nicotine in a traditional cigarette is delivered to the brain in 10 seconds when inhaled, but absorption ranges from minutes to hours when nicotine gum, lozenges, or patches are used.[43,44] There is no question that tobacco smoke and tobacco products are harmful.[45] However, a harm reduction debate exists in the public health community.[46] The associations between smoking and cancer and heart and lung disease are well-known and established among both smokers and nonsmokers. However, the health effects of other tobacco products, such as electronic cigarettes, are not as widely known, among both the public and scientists.[7]

Just as harmful effects of cigarettes took many years to discover, the relative safety or harm of the myriad of new tobacco products entering the market under the guise of harm reduction will take time to determine. Mass-produced and mass-marketed cigarettes were a 20th century experiment on the public health that has impacted the world like no other product before or after their development. Cigarettes are the single leading cause of preventable death, and an urgent response to the public health crisis is needed.[47]

The US Surgeon General has clearly stated that no safe level of exposure to tobacco smoke exists,[45] but limited scientific research is available on the safety of the vapor from e-cigarettes. Nor has adequate scientific research been performed on the effects of nicotine and the other chemicals in e-cigarette cartridges. E-cigarette advocates and manufacturers market the product as safer than conventional cigarette smoking. However, more research is needed to determine the safety and efficacy of e-cigarettes.

The e-cigarette industry has much to gain financially by promoting the harm reduction message.[11] Most smokers want to quit and many have tried without ultimate success, but smoking rates remain disproportionately high for some segments of the population.[48] E-cigarettes are an attractive option when coupled with a message of being less harmful, particularly as the cost of cigarettes and smoke-free environments continues to increase. Nonindustry studies are beginning to explore the effects of e-cigarette use on health and smoking cessation, but current findings are far from conclusive.[38,49] Despite the lack of research, sales of electronic cigarettes continue to rise.

Tobacco cessation experts cite the need for sound scientific studies, not market-driven data, to explore the potential efficacy of e-cigarettes or similar devices in helping people quit smoking.[4] If these devices can be shown to help more people quit completely, this would represent a true reduction of harm for users and the population as a whole. However, no scientific basis currently exists for making claims of either reduced harm or safety for e-cigarettes. Furthermore, e-cigarette use has potential unintended consequences, such as youth appeal, leading to increased smoking initiation, or dual use of different tobacco products by a single user, derailing the potential for ultimate smoking abstinence.

## OTHER CONCERNS

Henningfield and Zaatari[22] suggest that e-cigarettes may undermine smoke-free laws, cessation attempts, and prevention efforts. Specific concerns include (1) nicotine absorption does not mimic that of cigarettes and therefore e-cigarettes may not help smokers quit, (2) claims of safety to the user or to others breathing the emissions have not been verified; and (3) products delivering very low levels of nicotine may become "starter products" for nonsmokers, especially youth. Yamin and colleagues[4] elaborated on concerns for youth and young adults, a population that may respond to e-cigarettes being marketed as "green" and "healthy." Young children may be at high risk for toxicity from flavored cartridge refills containing lethal doses of nicotine.[4,34] Cahn and Siegel,[50] who support e-cigarettes as a promising harm reduction product, acknowledge that existing research does not establish the absolute safety of e-cigarettes. Additionally, concerns about abuse liability have been raised. Although very few participants used e-cigarettes for the delivery of other substances, a YouTube video shows how to refill the cartridge with marijuana hash oil.[5,36]

## REGULATORY AND POLICY ISSUES

Trtchounian and Talbot[23] evaluated five brands of e-cigarettes, finding potentially serious hazards in design, labeling, and print materials supplied with products or online; some examples follow. Cartridges leaked, and spent cartridges still contained liquid with dangerous nicotine. Loading cartridges may lead to dermal nicotine exposure, and nicotine-containing liquid from spent cartridges may leak onto surfaces, where carcinogens can form from exposure to air. Cartridge labels did not clearly communicate the amount of nicotine or the expiration date, nor any warnings about nicotine. Other issues included dead batteries, incorrect flashing codes, incorrect filling of orders, and inaccurate instructions and advertisements. A pervasive lack of quality control exists in the manufacturing, marketing, and distribution of e-cigarettes.

The WHO calls for the study of pharmacokinetics, safety and efficacy trials, and approval by drug regulatory agencies.[51] Studies would include a complete description of the ingredients, concentrations of chemicals delivered to the consumer, comparisons of cessation outcomes, and identification of adverse effects. Yamin and colleagues[4] call for monitoring of biologic, social, and addictive effects and of online promotions of e-cigarettes. WHO further recommends that national health surveys monitor e-cigarette use and that practitioners counsel patients against using e-cigarettes.[51]

Henningfield and Zaatari[22] concur with the WHO's recommendation that e-cigarettes be covered under smoke-free laws and tobacco-free policies. Without evidence that e-cigarettes and their emissions are safe, increasing numbers of agencies, companies, and governments are including e-cigarette use in their smoke-free policies. For example, the Air Force and the Marine base at Quantico prohibit use of e-cigarettes in the workplace, and New Jersey and Suffolk County, NY, prohibit their use wherever smoking is prohibited.[52] The US Department of Transportation now applies the federal regulation against smoking on aircraft to e-cigarettes.[12] Canada, Australia, Brazil, and Panama have prohibited e-cigarettes entirely because of safety and regulatory concerns.[4] King County, Wash, and Tacoma Wash, limit e-cigarette use inside public places[12] and four Kentucky communities prohibit use of e-cigarettes in public places and workplaces.[53] Six states and six communities prohibit e-cigarette sales to minors.[12] Americans for Nonsmokers' Rights urges university campuses to prohibit use of e-cigarettes as a part of their tobacco-free campus policies.[54]

## RESEARCH AGENDA

The scarce scientific evidence available indicates that toxic and carcinogenic compounds are present in e-cigarettes, although in lower concentrations than in traditional cigarettes. Actual contents vary widely, even among e-cigarettes of the same label, and the labeling does not always reflect the contents. More rigorous chemical analyses are needed, as are animal studies and clinical trials in humans to test the safety and efficacy of e-cigarettes.[2]

Standardization of the products and regulation of manufacturing practices are needed before research can be conducted. Otherwise, the variability in cartridge and vapor content may jeopardize study results, minimizing generalizability.[7] As of September 2011, e-cigarettes were marketed legally in the United States without clinical trials, and the companies developing them were not likely to have the resources for adequate testing. As a precondition for safety and efficacy research on e-cigarettes, Etter and colleagues[7] call for an urgent need to develop resources for testing and a legal framework in which manufacturers are licensed and accountable to manufacturing regulations. Without this standardization, the rapidly evolving e-cigarette technology means new products constantly arrive on the market, making research obsolete at the time of publication. Applying this legal framework not only has the potential to remove unsafe products from the market but also may contribute to the safety and efficacy of new smoking cessation drugs and devices that could save lives.[7] Unfortunately, the United States seems to be in the middle of another grand experiment on the public's health, driven by the marketplace rather than science.

## SUMMARY AND NURSING IMPLICATIONS

Hundreds of small companies produce e-cigarettes, which are not currently regulated in the United States as drugs or drug delivery devices. Based on a recent court decision, the FDA can and will regulate e-cigarettes as tobacco products (unless marketed as making therapeutic claims) and less scrutiny will be applied, despite preliminary findings that they contain toxic ingredients varying widely among and within brands. Furthermore, consumers are not adequately informed because the ingredients may not be represented accurately on the label. Even if companies do not officially market e-cigarettes as cessation aids, numerous online consumer testimonies give the impression that e-cigarettes can help smokers quit and that use of e-cigarettes should be permitted anywhere. Some authors have supported the use of e-cigarettes, citing harm reduction as the rationale, despite the dearth of evidence about what the cartridges or vapor contain or whether the products are safe or effective. Design and manufacturing issues further exacerbate safety concerns for users and their families. Very little is known about e-cigarette emissions and no standardized way to study the vapor is available. Many authors call for further research, but standardization of the product and its manufacture is needed before research findings can be generalized beyond a particular brand and batch of e-cigarettes. Funding is needed for non–industry-sponsored research, because most small companies do not have the resources. However, the potential exists to add another well-tested, safe, and effective cessation product to the public health arsenal. As Etter and colleagues[7] suggest, sound research would form empiric bases for decisions made by regulators, elected officials, health care providers, and consumers.

Kuschner and colleagues[19] recommend that clinicians inform patients that e-cigarettes are not approved as cessation devices by the FDA and that no evidence supports that they help smokers quit. The investigators urge clinicians to use strategies recommended by the Public Health Service–sponsored Clinical Practice Guideline[41] and the telephone quitlines: 1-800-QUIT-NOW. Cobb and Abrams[5] concur, also recommending that patients wishing to use nicotine as a quit strategy be directed to one of the many FDA-regulated and safe forms of nicotine replacement, along with other effective tools, such as Web-based services. Kuschner and colleagues[19] further suggest informing clients that using e-cigarettes may give children and teens the impression that "vaping" is harmless. The authors also note that millions of people (more than half of ever-smokers alive today) have achieved long-term abstinence.[19] In conclusion, nurses need to direct tobacco users to evidence-based quit strategies and cessation products; support inclusion of e-cigarettes in smoke-free policies and prohibiting sales to minors; and advocate for further research and surveillance of the use and marketing of e-cigarettes.

## ACKNOWLEDGMENTS

The authors acknowledge the clinical and intellectual contributions of Kelly Owens at the Madison County Health Department in Richmond, Kentucky, and Rachel Grana at the Center for Tobacco Control Research & Education, University of California San Francisco.

## REFERENCES

1. FDA and public health experts warn about electronic cigarettes. U.S. Food and Drug Association Web site. Available at: http://www.fda.gov/NewsEvents/ Newsroom/PressAnnouncements/ucm173222.htm. Accessed October 19, 2010.
2. Flouris AD, Oikonomou DN. Electronic cigarettes: miracle or menace. Personal view. BMJ 2010;340:215.
3. Eissenberg T. Electronic nicotine delivery devices: ineffective nicotine delivery and craving suppression after acute administration [letters]. Tob Control 2010; 19(1):87–8.
4. Yamin CK, Bitton A, Bates DW. E-cigarettes: a rapidly growing Internet phenomenon. Ann Intern Med 2010;153(9):607–9.
5. Cobb NK, Abrams DB. E-cigarette or drug-delivery device? Regulating novel nicotine products. N Engl J Med 2011;365(3):193–5.
6. McQueen A, Tower S, Sumner W. Interviews with "vapers": implications for future research with electronic cigarettes. Nicotine Tob Res 2011;13(9):860–7.
7. Etter JF, Bullen C, Flouris AD. Electronic nicotine delivery systems: a research agenda. Tob Control 2011;20(3):243–8.
8. Rodu B. The scientific foundation for tobacco harm reduction, 2006-2011. Harm Reduct J 2011;8(9).
9. E-cigarettes: questions and answers. U.S. Food and Drug Administration Web site. Available at: http://www.fda.gov/ForConsumers/ConsumerUpdates/ucm225 210.htm. Accessed August 20, 2011.
10. Pauly J, Qiang L, Barry MB. Tobacco-free electronic cigarettes and cigars deliver nicotine and generate concern. Tob Control 2007;16:357.
11. Noel JK, Rees VW, Connolly GN. Electronic cigarettes: a new 'tobacco' industry? Tob Control 2011;20:81.
12. Electronic cigarettes: how they are—and could be—regulated. Public Health Law & Policy Technical Assistance Legal Center Web site. Available at: http: //www.phlpnet.org/sites/phlpnet.org/files/7-03_e-cigarette_FactSht4.pdf. Accessed August 21, 2011.
13. Kuehn BM. Health agencies update. Regulation for e-cigarettes. JAMA 2010; 304(10):1777.
14. Kirshner L. Recent case developments. Am J Law Med 2011;37:194–8.
15. Regulation of e-cigarettes and other tobacco products. Letter to stakeholders. U.S. Food and Drug Administration Web site. Available at: http://www.fda.gov/ NewsEvents/PublicHealthFocus/ucm252360.htm. Accessed August 20, 2011.
16. Kesmodel D, Yadron D. E-cigarettes spark new smoking war. Available at: http:// online.wsj.com. Accessed July 15, 2011.
17. Swedberg C. Manufacturing news. RFID makes matches for e-cigarette smokers. RFID Journal Web site. Available at: http://www.rfidjournal.com/ article/view/8471. Accessed August 25, 2011.
18. Grana RA, Glantz SA, Ling PM. Industry watch. Electronic nicotine delivery systems in the hands of Hollywood. Tob Control 2011.
19. Kuschner WG, Reddy S, Mehrotra N. Electronic cigarettes and thirdhand tobacco smoke: two emerging health care challenges for the primary care provider. Int J Gen Med 2011;4:115–20.

20. Research on management of electronic cigarette. National Evidence-based Healthcare Collaborating Agency Web site. Available at: http://cfile10.uf.tistory. com/attach/2028135A4D242B9B174B8B. Accessed August 13, 2011.

21. Benowitz NL. Cigarette smoking and cardiovascular disease: pathophysiology and implications for treatment. Prog Cardiovasc Dis 2003;46(1):91–111.

22. Henningfield JE, Zaatari GS. Electronic nicotine delivery systems: Emerging science foundation for policy. Tob Control 2010;19(2):89–90.

23. Trtchounian A, Talbot P. Electronic nicotine delivery systems: is there a need for regulation? Tob Control 2011;20:47–52.

24. Sleiman MA, Gundel LA, Pankow JF, et al. Formation of carcinogens indoors by surface-mediated reactions of nicotine with nitrous acid, leading to potential thirdhand smoke hazards. Proc Natl Acad Sci U S A 2010;107(15):6576–81.

25. Westenberger BJ. Evaluation of e-cigarettes. U.S. Food and Drug Association Web site. 2009. Available at: http://www.fda.gov/downloads/Drugs/ScienceResearch/ UCM173250.pdf. Accessed August 22, 2011.

26. Hadwiger ME, Trehy ML, Ye W, et al. Identification of amino-tadalafil and rimonabant in electronic cigarette products using high pressure liquid chromatography with diode array and tandem mass spectrometric detection. J Chromatogr A 2010;1217:7547–55.

27. A guide to glycols. Dow Chemical Company Web site. Available at: http://www.dow. com/PublishedLiterature/dh_02aa/09002f13802aaf25.pdf. Accessed September 5, 2011.

28. Varughese S, Teschke K, Brauer M, et al. Effects of theatrical smokes and fogs on respiratory health in the entertainment industry. Am J Ind Med 2005;47: 411–8.

29. Propylene glycol information update: considerations against use in theatrical fogs. American Chemistry Council Web site. Available at: http://www.dow.com/Published Literature/dh_0047/0901b803800479d9.pdf#page=36. Accessed August 14, 2011.

30. Montharu J, Le Guellec S, Kittel B, et al. Evaluation of lung tolerance of ethanol, propylene glycol, and sorbitan monooleate as solvents in medical aerosols. J Aerosol Med Pulm Drug Deliv 2010;23(1):41–6.

31. Werley MS, McDonald P, Lilly P, et al. Non-clinical safety and pharmacokinetic evaluations of propylene glycol aerosol in Sprague-Dawley rats and Beagle dogs. Toxicology 2011;287:76–90.

32. Schep LJ, Slaughter RJ, Temple WA, et al. Diethylene glycol poisoning. Clin Toxicol 2009;47(6):525–35.

33. Laugesen M. Safety report on the Ruyan® e-cigarette cartridge and inhaled aerosol. Christchurch (New Zealand): Health New Zealand Ltd; 2008.

34. Etter JF. Electronic cigarettes: a survey of users. BMC Public Health 2010;10:231.

35. Siegel MB, Tanwar KL, Wood KS. Electronic cigarettes as a smoking-cessation tool. Am J Prev Med 2011;40(4):472–5.

36. Etter JF, Bullen C. Electronic cigarette: users profile, utilization, satisfaction and perceived efficacy. Addiction 2011;106(11):2017–28.

37. Capponetto P, Polosa R, Auditore R, et al. Smoking cessation with e-cigarettes in smokers with a documented history of depression and recurring relapses. Int J Clin Med 2011;2:281–4.

38. Bullen C, McRobbie H, Thornley S, et al. Effect of an electronic nicotine delivery device (e-cigarette) on desire to smoke and withdrawal, user preferences and nicotine delivery: randomised cross-over trial. Tob Control 2010;19(2):98–103.

39. Vansickel AR, Cobb CO, Weaver MF, et al. A clinical laboratory model for evaluating the acute effects of electronic "cigarettes": nicotine delivery profile and

cardiovascular and subjective effects. Cancer Epidemiol Biomarkers Prev 2011; 19:1945.

40. Trtchounian A, Williams M, Talbot P. Conventional and electronic cigarettes (e-cigarettes) have different smoking characteristics. Nicotine Tob Res 2010; 12(9):905–12.

41. Fiore MC, Jaen CR, Baker TB, et al. Treating tobacco use and dependence: 2008 update. Rockville (MD): U.S. Department of Health and Human Services; 2008.

42. Shiffman S, Brockwell SE, Pillitteri JL, et al. Use of smoking-cessation treatments in the United States. Am J Prev Med 2008;34(2):102–11.

43. Benowitz NL. Pharmacology of nicotine: addiction, smoking-induced disease, and therapeutics. Annu Rev Pharmacol Toxicol 2009;49:57–71.

44. Picciotto MR, Corrigall WA. Neuronal systems underlying behaviors related to nicotine addiction: neural circuits and molecular genetics. J Neurosci 2002; 22(9):3338–41.

45. U.S. Department of Health and Human Services. How tobacco smoke causes disease: the biology and behavioral basis for smoking-attributable disease: a report of the Surgeon General. Atlanta (GA): U.S. Department of Health and Human Services, Centers for Disease Control and Prevention, National Center for Chronic Disease Prevention and Health Promotion, Office on Smoking and Health; 2010.

46. Zeller M, Hatsukami D. The Strategic Dialogue on Tobacco Harm Reduction: a vision and blueprint for action in the US. Tob Control 2009;18(4):324–32.

47. Beaglehole R, Bonita R, Horton R, et al. Priority actions for the non-communicable disease crisis. Lancet 2011;378(9791):565.

48. Garrett BE, Dube SR, Trosclair A, et al. Cigarette smoking - United States, 1965-2008. MMWR Surveill Summ 2011;60(Suppl):109–13.

49. Foulds J, Veldheer S, Berg A. Electronic cigarettes (e-cigs): views of aficionados and clinical/public health perspectives. Int J Clin Pract 2011;65(10):1037–42.

50. Cahn S, Siegel M. Electronic cigarettes as a harm reduction strategy for tobacco control: a step forward or a repeat of past mistakes? J Public Health Policy 2011; 32:6–31.

51. World Health Organization. Regulatory scope. Tobacco product regulation. Electronic nicotine delivery systems. Drug Information 2010;24(1):30–2. Available at: http://www.who.int/medicines/publications/druginformation/DrugInfo2010_Vol24-1.pdf. Accessed August 20, 2011.

52. E-cigarettes banned on domestic flights, reports ASH. Action on Smoking and Health (ASH) Web site. Available at: http://www.prlog.org/10942504-cigarettes-banned-on-domestic-flights-reports-ash.html. Accessed October 19, 2010.

53. Smoke-free ordinances and regulations in Kentucky. Kentucky Center for Smoke-free Policy Web site. Available at: http://www.mc.uky.edu/TobaccoPolicy/KCSP/. Accessed September 2, 2011.

54. Model policy for a smokefree university. Americans for Nonsmokers' Rights Web site. Available at: http://www.no-smoke.org/pdf/modeluniversitypolicy.pdf. Accessed August 29, 2011.

# Index

*Note:* Page numbers of article titles are in **boldface** type.

Nurs Clin N Am 47 (2012) 173–179
doi:10.1016/S0029-6465(12)00017-5
0029-6465/12/$ – see front matter © 2012 Elsevier Inc. All rights reserved.

nursing.theclinics.com

# Moving?

## Make sure your subscription moves with you!

To notify us of your new address, find your **Clinics Account Number** (located on your mailing label above your name), and contact customer service at:

**Email: journalscustomerservice-usa@elsevier.com**

**800-654-2452** (subscribers in the U.S. & Canada)
**314-447-8871** (subscribers outside of the U.S. & Canada)

**Fax number: 314-447-8029**

**Elsevier Health Sciences Division**
**Subscription Customer Service**
**3251 Riverport Lane**
**Maryland Heights, MO 63043**

*To ensure uninterrupted delivery of your subscription, please notify us at least 4 weeks in advance of move.

ELSEVIER